"Bakalinsky . . . is the Ferdinand Magellan, the Sir Francis
Drake, the Vasco da Gama of San Francisco stairways."

—Paul McHugh, *San Francisco Chronicle*

". . . a fascinating trek through the sidewalk staircases hidden
around the city."

—*The New York Times*

". . . a wonderfully informative guidebook, custom-made for
a city with challenging hills and picture-perfect views . . .
chock full of fascinating details . . ."

—*Travel Books Review*

"Bakalinsky has been scouring the city since the mid-1970s,
clambering, walking, exploring tiny alleys and stairways,
grand steps, paths and risers that interlace the city."

—*San Diego Union-Tribune*

"Bakalinsky. . . is the reigning queen of walkers in a city
that's full of them."

—Joe Yonan, *The Washington Post*

*Everything of importance has already been seen
by somebody who didn't notice it.*
                                    —Alfred North Whitehead

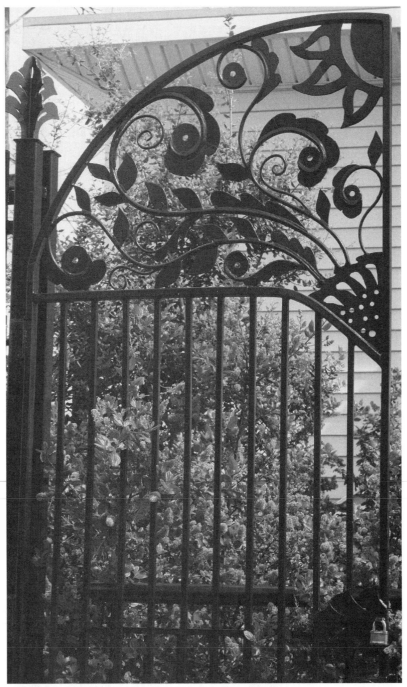

Visitacion Valley Greenway Herb Garden (Walk 26) *Annette Hovie*

Stairway Walks in San Francisco

The Joy of Urban Exploring

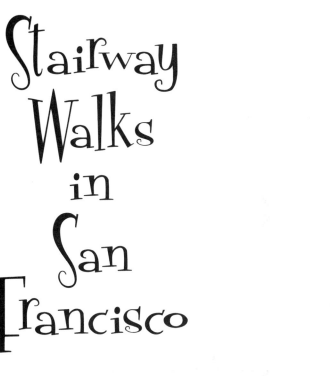

Adah Bakalinsky

with Marian Gregoire

WILDERNESS PRESS ... *on the trail since 1967*

Stairway Walks in San Francisco

3rd EDITION April 1995
4th EDITION September 2001
5th EDITION April 2004
6th EDITION January 2007
7th EDITION 2010
  3rd printing 2012

Cover and interior photos copyright © 2010 by their respective photographers
Maps: Ben Pease, Charles Brock, and Marian Gregoire
Cover and interior design: Larry B. Van Dyke
Editor: Laura Shauger
Indexer: Rich Carlson

ISBN 978-0-89997-637-2

Manufactured in the United States

Published by: **Wilderness Press**
               Keen Communications
               PO Box 43673
               Birmingham, AL 35243
               (800) 443-7227; FAX (205) 326-1012
               www.wildernesspress.com

Visit our website for a complete listing of our books and ordering information.

Distributed by Publishers Group West

Cover photos: (Clockwise from upper left) Coit Tower (Peter Nagy), mosaic tile
  stairway at 16th Ave. and Moraga in Golden Gate Heights (James Charney),
  and Vulcan Stairway in Upper Market (Tony Holiday)

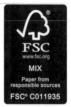

SAFETY NOTICE: Although Wilderness Press and the author
have made every attempt to ensure that the information in this
book is accurate at press time, they are not responsible for any
loss, damage, injury, or inconvenience that may occur to anyone while using this book. You are responsible for your own
safety and health. The fact that a stairway walk is described in
this book does not mean that it will be safe for you. Be aware
that conditions can change from day to day. Use good judg-
ment and minimize your risk on any stairway walk or urban
hike by being knowledgeable, prepared, and alert.

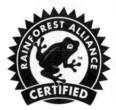

Dedication

I dedicate the seventh edition of *Stairway Walks in San Francisco* to a three-part wish:

> that all children discover the spirit and joy of walking and exploring the City's neighborhoods;

> that all children develop an appreciation and awareness that nature and man-made beauty can exist in harmony;

> that all children throughout their lives will become stewards and actively contribute to the livability of the cities where they live.

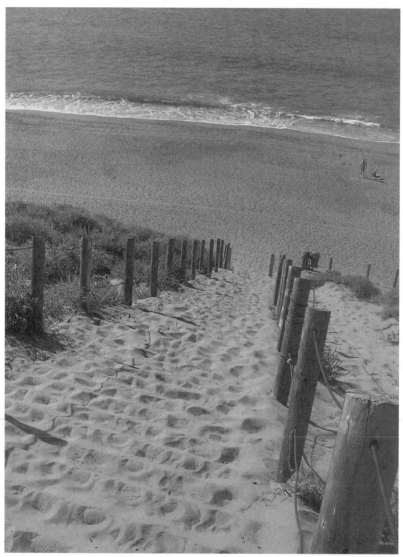

Sand ladder at Baker Beach

Tony Holiday

Contents

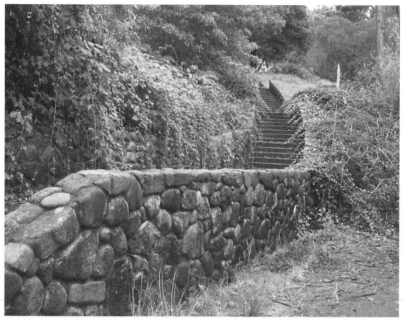

A stairway in Fort Scott (Walk 9)

Adah Bakalinsky

Acknowledgments

I feel favored to live in San Francisco. It is the perfect place for me to continue the tradition of walking that I enjoyed with my parents and grandparents. I never tire of exploring the neighborhoods and walking the hills. I always find someone to talk with who shares another portion of San Francisco history with me. Plus I enjoy the weather.

I feel favored to have so many people to thank for their share in *Stairway Walks in San Francisco*. Beginning with the first edition, I found one person and then another and another who offered advice, assistance with maps, drawings, editorial work, or route checking. The list has grown longer with each edition—only a scroll could accommodate it. Therefore, this seventh edition lists those persons principally involved with the present effort. Many of these people I originally met on my walks.

I thank the adventuresome friends who at short notice were available for consultation and on-site forays: Michael Lampen, a third-generation native San Franciscan, is an excellent historian and geologist who, over the years, has been my generous source of definitive information. Niki Goldsborough is always ready to share her love of plants. Mary Burk shares her ideas and knowledge of what's going on in the world of technology. Damien Raffa has always returned calls regarding ongoing developments at the Presidio Trust. Tony Holiday, ever curious, is always ready to check out an esoteric house, alley, or stairway, and share his photos. Peter Ehrlich, chief forester of the Presidio Trust, allowed me to record his enthusiastic and detailed story of the installation of Andy Goldsworthy's 100-foot-tall *Spire* in the Presidio. Isabel Wade (now retired) and her extraordinary staff at Neighborhood Parks Alliance made a special birthday walk for my two-week-old great-grandchild a reality. She introduced me to the Blue Greenway, and its informed advocate, Corinne Woods.

I see our neighborhoods and open spaces from another point of view when friends from outside the San Francisco area come to walk and explore them. Berkeley residents Paul Grunland and Jacque Ensign love the Lands End walk. Dick Farrar from Rancho Palo Verde can complete two neighborhood walks in one day using public transportation to connect him to the starting point. Before Laury Bird leaves for his home in Santa Monica, he spends his last San Francisco morning exploring a neighborhood. Roger Mansfield of Colorado Springs, in one day, managed to meet with fellow astronomers at the Planetarium, walked a section of Golden Gate Heights, and completed the day hiking Lands End. Bregtje Schudel from Holland on her way to Japan and England, spent her two days here exploring Golden Gate Heights and the Twin Peaks neighborhoods. Lonna Necker and Mary Farha and their group of walkers from Sonoma County have been coming once a month since 2007 to explore San Francisco neighborhood pathways. Ethan Baker from Thousand Oaks walked up the Greenwich Stairway to Coit Tower, 388 stairs, and walked down the Greenwich Stairway to Sansome, 388 stairs, when he was five years old.

I am also gratified to hear stories of local people who regularly walk neighborhoods with friends and make the activity a social event. Sandy Michelotti and her friend have been doing this for years, and through their enthusiasm and gifts of the stairways book have encouraged others to explore and enjoy San Francisco neighborhoods.

I rely on neighborhood informants for their news about the planning stage, the problems, and the successes. Neighborhoods are the heart of the City, and when they're healthy, we all share the health. Thanks to Alice Yee, Howard Munson, Judy Irving, Fran Martin, and Mark Ryser.

Leonardo da Vinci said, "Feet are masterpieces of engineering." To that observation I add: Fit feet promote soaring spirits, a winning combination for urban walking and exploring. My hearty thanks to William Jenkin, my podiatrist, who has been encouraging me to continue my walking and exploring style, and is alert to any mischievous intent among my toes and their connected relatives.

I mumble special wordless thanks (because I don't know the words to express my undying gratitude) to two people whose DNA are linked to stairways and urban exploring. Charles Brock, Marian Gregoire, and I have worked together on the sixth and seventh editions of the book. Even though Charles has moved out of the area, he assists with stairway cataloging and text and map proofing. Marian Gregoire has worked with me, tirelessly, on the seventh edition. The three of us bounce ideas off each other, inspiring new ideas and revisions of ideas. Both of them have a perfect sense of direction. I counterbalance them.

Thanks to Kate Brock, James Charney, Polly Gates, Tony Holiday, Annette Hovie, Clayton Juan, Peter Nagy, Presidio Trust, and Peter Wanger for sharing their photos. A special thanks to Polly Gates, my eldest daughter, whom I've known since day one, whose candor and insistence on clarity of expression demanded focus, restraint, and refreshment of imagination on my part. Throughout the years I have collected quotations and anecdotes about walking, in anticipation of hosting an imaginary dinner party, attended by people who were noted everyday walkers. They poetically express themselves about the art of urban exploration, lively conversations ensue, and a splendid time is had by all. Some of the quotations are scattered throughout the book.

A thousand thanks to one and all.

Foreword

Back in the days when I was living on the street, I survived by doing various odd jobs. One of the most common was cleaning houses. I made a habit of perusing the library in every house I cleaned, and I nearly always found a copy of *Stairway Walks in San Francisco* on the shelves. For some reason it grabbed my attention. Maybe because the author had such an interesting sounding name. Or maybe because I never got out of the City and I saw the book as a portal to exotic locations that were within my reach.

I knew a few of the stairways in the book—the ones on Russian Hill and Telegraph Hill—and they were among my favorite routes. I always envied those fortunate enough to live there, and never imagined I'd end up being among them. In 1988, I moved onto the Greenwich Steps, and, except for one year, I've been here ever since. This is where I met the wild parrot flock that changed my life.

For a long time my friendship with the birds was a private affair that only neighbors and the occasional passersby knew anything about. Then one day, I heard a knock on my door and found Adah Bakalinsky standing on my porch. While giving a guided tour of the Greenwich Steps, she'd seen me feeding the parrots. She wanted to know whether I had any slides of the birds. I said, "Well, yes. A lot." Adah said she'd like to set up some slide shows for me. I was reluctant, but she asked so sweetly that I managed only a feeble protest. Those shows changed everything. Because of them I wrote a book. I also met my wife, Judy Irving, who made a popular movie about me and my crazy-winged friends.

All this happened because Adah pays close attention to and nurtures the worlds she writes about in her book. Read it, follow the tours, and discover the hidden corners of the real San Francisco. You never know what might happen.

—*Mark Bittner*

Mark Bittner is the author of *The Wild Parrots of Telegraph Hill*, the basis for the documentary of the same name by Judy Irving. Mark and Judy live on Telegraph Hill.

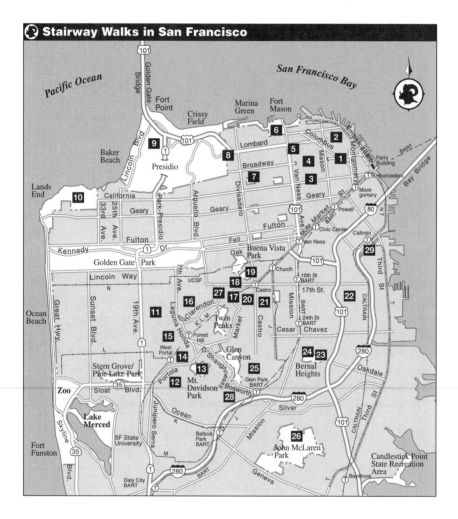

Stairway Walks in San Francisco

LIST OF STAIRWAY WALKS

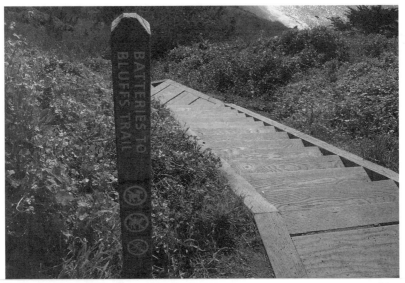

Batteries to Bluff Stairway (Walk 9)   *Tony Holiday*

Introduction

Those of us who love stairways cherish the
image of the unknown walker of eons ago, who,
walking in the indentations on the sides of the cliff,
visualized them as a welcome shortcut up the hill. Exer-
cising ingenuity and mathematical skill, this walker developed the principle of comfortable stairways. Jacques François
Blondel in his 1771 *Cours d'Architecture* was the first known person to establish the ergonomic relationship of tread to riser dimen-
sions. He specified that two times riser plus tread equals 26 inches.
I love neighborhoods. They are the heart and soul of a city. I have
become cognizant of ways that residents of a community become
neighbors. They focus on a communal problem. Stairways serve as
an essential focal point for people to work together, either to repair a
stairway, to plant flowers and shrubs on the sides of stairways, or to
embellish a stairway. In the beginning of my adventures around the
neighborhoods, I had no idea that stairways were an important aspect
of urban design and an integrating feature for community organization. They provide open space for walkers to walk freely without
the threat of cars behind them. People can sit on the stairs, visit with
friends, or talk with persons who do become friends (that happens to
me all the time). I have a file of stairway stories—love stories, communal work stories, and friendship stories. In all of them the stairway
is the catalyst that brings people together. Stairways also provide a
conduit between neighborhoods that allow a pedestrian to expand a
walk through two or three of them. Stairways connect neighborhoods;
freeways disconnect neighborhoods.

Neighborhoods go through cycles of declining, decaying, recover-
ing, and blooming. Stairways are an indicator artifact; they tell the
condition of the neighborhood. One of the most satisfying aspects
of urban exploring and stairway walking is talking with neighbors
and sharing what I learn from one group with another working on

a similar problem. The idealism, the energy, and the commitment to their community are all there. With assistance and encouragement from San Francisco Beautiful, the foremost local nonprofit since 1947 dedicated to creating, enhancing, and protecting the livability of San Francisco, we have added beauty to various parts of the City—the mosaic tile stairway in Golden Gate Heights, one of the most beautiful stairways in the country; the new stairway/gardens in Bernal Heights East; the Pemberton brick-shaped, terracotta, concrete stairway in the Twin Peaks neighborhood that was a welcome aesthetic challenge for the city designers; and the new stairways around Pioneer Park and Coit Tower.

San Francisco is a "walking city." Built upon 42 hills, it is surrounded by the Bay on the east, the Pacific on the west, a peninsula on the south, and on the north, the Golden Gate. Within those confines, variety is constant. Light and water combine to produce striking effects on bridges and buildings throughout the day; at sunset, the beams of light dramatize the hills, sides of houses, and the mirrors in the mosaic stairway at Moraga and 16th Avenue.

The hills accelerate changes in perspective as one walks around corners or circles the ridges. Landmarks recede and suddenly emerge in a landscape abounding in inclines and angled streets. The Mt. Sutro TV tower viewed from the mid-Sunset District is a beautiful sky sculpture; from the Sutro area, it looks like a ship in space. From Ashbury Heights, it looks pedestrian. It appears large and within touching distance from the Outer Sunset District; walk two blocks toward it, and it appears distant and small.

The streets of San Francisco range from comparatively flat, such as Irving, to almost vertical, such as sections of Duboce, Filbert, and Duncan. In fact, the City fathers and developers found grading the streets a primary obstacle in converting San Francisco from a tent town into a city of timbered houses. Some of the hills were completely demolished in the process; others were cut into without much planning. When the task seemed insurmountable, the "street" ended. That's why we have many triangles and other odd shapes left over, sparking neighbors to cooperate and establish mini-gardens.

How does one maneuver from one street level to another when there are so many hills? Via stairways, of course! There are more than 670 stairways of all descriptions: crooked, straight, short, long, concrete, wood, balustraded, unadorned, narrow, and wide. Our streets were pummeled and pushed into rectangular grids familiar from the East Coast, but inappropriate to our terrain. Paved streets often follow the contours of hills, but the stairways allow a direct vertical approach from one street to another. They provide accessibility to public transportation; they provide safety in case of fire; and they limit degradation of the land. Plus everyone loves a shortcut.

The 29 walks in the book vary in length and elevation. They are designed for the curious walker who loves to explore. Each walk takes between two and two and a half hours if you enjoy all the sights, scents, and sounds along the way. I have included walks in familiar neighborhoods like Pacific Heights and Telegraph Hill and walks in less familiar neighborhoods like Eureka Valley and Edgehill. In all of them, I have found visual interest in the immediate setting and in the surrounding areas, and always, stories by neighbors.

The beginning point of each walk can be reached by public transportation (call 311 or visit www.sfmuni.com for routes and schedules) or the free PresidiGo shuttle for the Presidio, call (415) 561-5300 or visit www.presidio.gov/tenants/transit/downtown.htm. Buses are available at several points of most walks, and alternate routes are occasionally suggested for specific reasons. Some of the walks are quite strenuous, but the rewards of stupendous views and delightful discoveries justify the effort. In order to appreciate the scaffolding of the City and the variety of neighborhoods within a whistle's call, I've included some graceful links to other walks in other neighborhoods that can be traversed comfortably in a single session.

Map Legend

Featured Stairway	ııııııııııııııı	Start/End of Walk	
Featured Street	▬▬▬	Intermediate Points	
Featured Path	▬ ▬ ▬ ▬	Picnic Area	⊞
Alternate Route	·············	Building	▪
Other Stairway	ıııııııııııııı	Gate	↔
Other Path	─ ─ ─ ─ ─	Hill	▲
Street	══════	Address	200
Rail Transit Route and Station	┄┼┄Ⓣ┄	Park or Preserve	
North Arrow		Other Open Space	
		Body of Water	

I suggest walkers carry the following gear to make the adventure more comfortable: binoculars, a city map, a compass, water, fruit, and layered clothing, especially long pants and long-sleeved shirts for walks where vegetation may hide poison oak. I use the directions left and right, but also the compass points—north, east, south, and west—to provide additional assurance. I highly recommend the map, Nature in the City, which is available without charge from the Department of Recreation and Parks. It shows the parks and other green areas in the City. The Neighborhood Parks Alliance is the organization that promotes parks and open spaces. They hold scheduled volunteer workdays on a regular basis. The SF Green Schoolyard Alliance promotes school gardens where children work and learn botany and gardening skills through an integrated curriculum. This edition includes an up-to-date listing of every public stairway in San Francisco. Only one person in the world knows every public stairway and every step in every public stairway in San Francisco, and has walked every stairway, in new combinations of walks, not once, but many times—Charles Brock. His efforts doubled my previous list.

The descriptions in the walks were up-to-date at publication time. However, neighborhoods continually evolve. If you find discrepancies, please inform Wilderness Press.

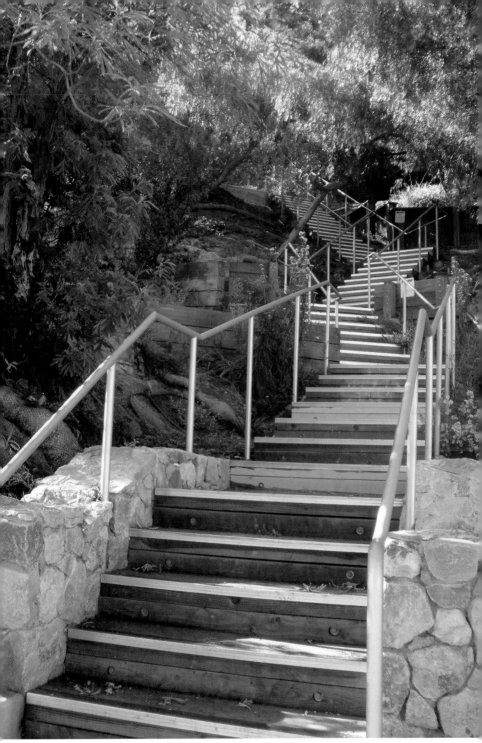

Buena Vista Park, Corona Heights (Walk 19)

Marion Gregoire

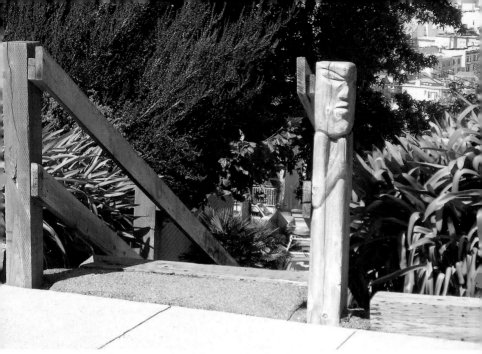

Franconia Stairway, Bernal Heights East (Walk 23) *Tony Holiday*

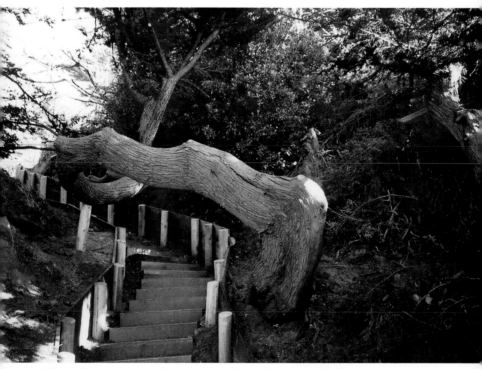

Mile Rock Stairway on the Coastal Trail, Lands End (Walk 10) *Peter Nagy*

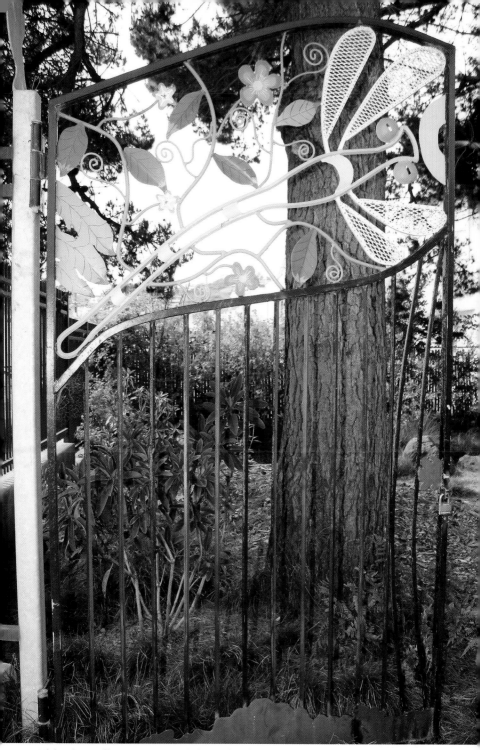

Visitacion Valley Greenway Herb Garden (Walk 26)

Annette Hovie

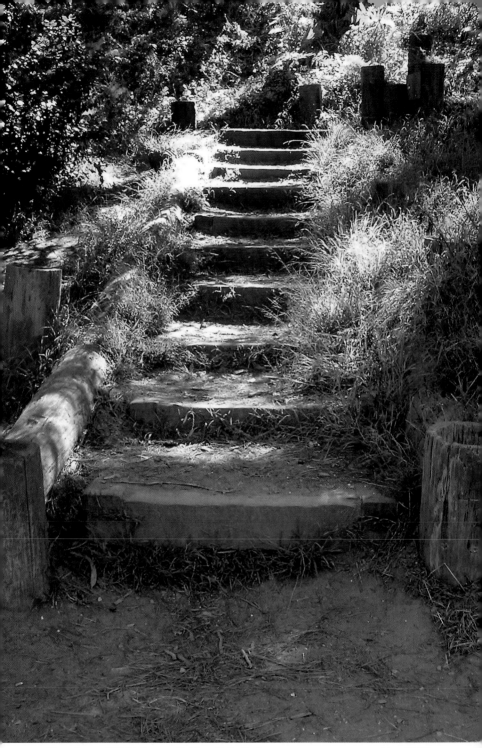

Strawberry Hill Stairway, Golden Gate Park

Tony Holiday

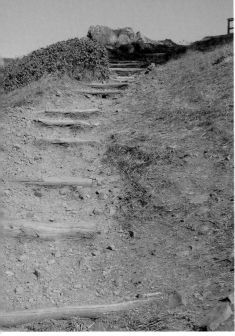

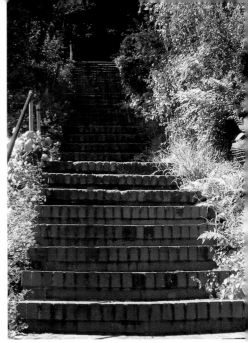

**Tank Hill Stairway, Twin Peaks
Foothills (Walk 17)** *Tony Holiday*

**Jack Early Park Stairway, Telegraph
Hill (Walk 2)** *Tony Holiday*

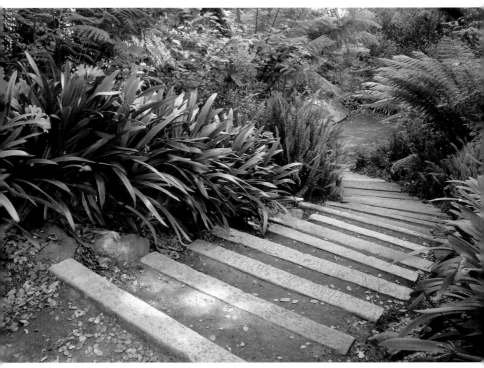

AIDS Memorial Grove Stairway, Golden Gate Park *Tony Holiday*

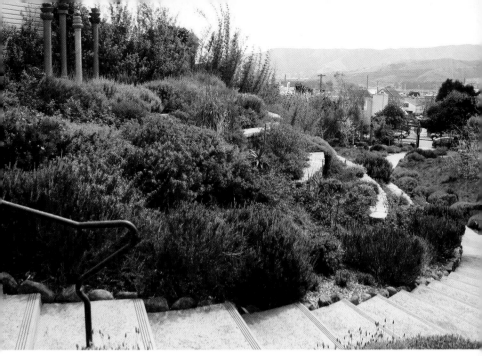

Visitacion Valley Greenway (Walk 26) *Annette Hovie*

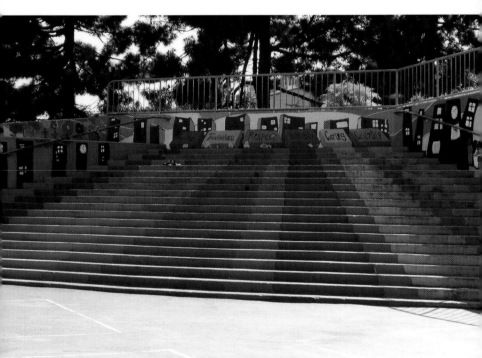

McKinley School Playground, Corona Heights (Walk 19) *Adah Bakalinsky*

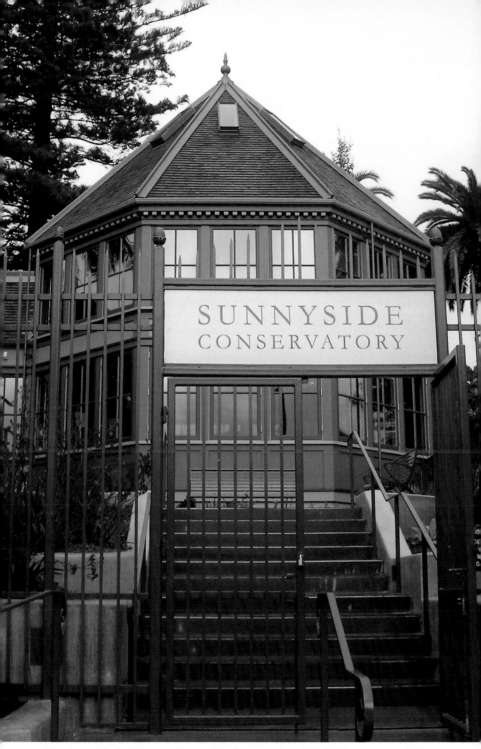

Monterey Blvd. Entrance, Sunnyside Conservatory (Walk 28)   *Tony Holiday*

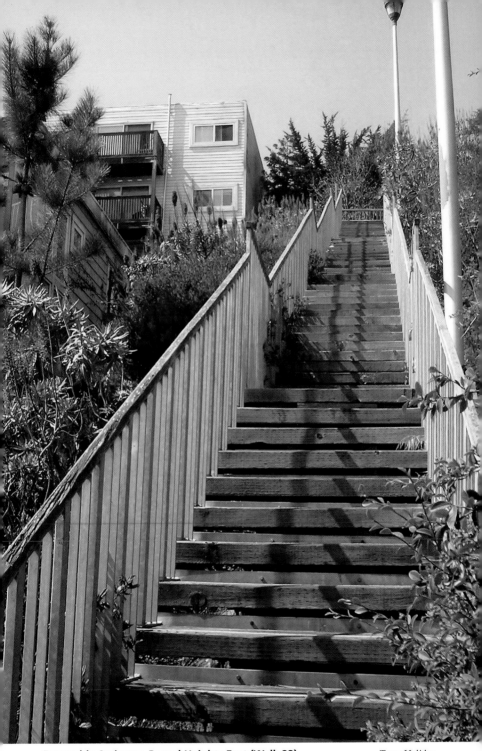

Esmeralda Stairway, Bernal Heights East (Walk 23)   *Tony Holiday*

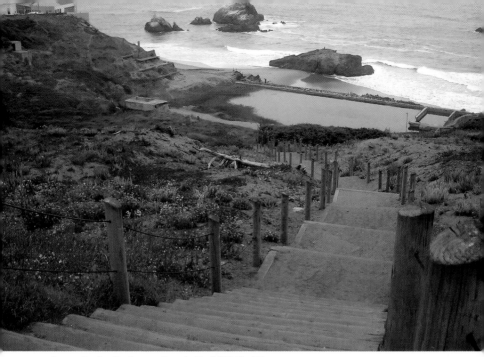

Sutro Baths Stairway, Lands End (Walk 10) *Tony Holiday*

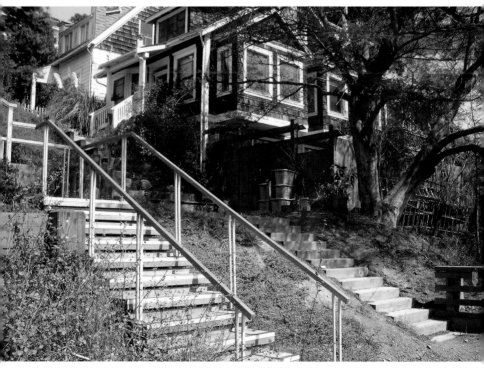

Powhattan Stairway, Bernal Heights West (Walk 24) *Tony Holi-*

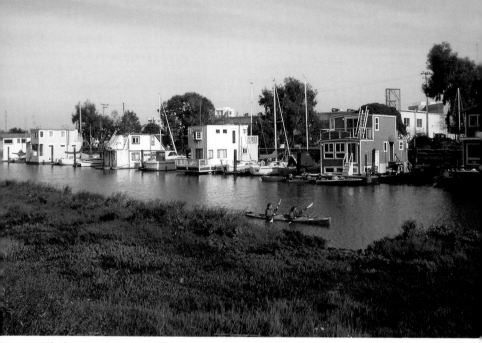

Mission Creek Marina, The Blue Greenway (Walk 29) *Tony Holi-*

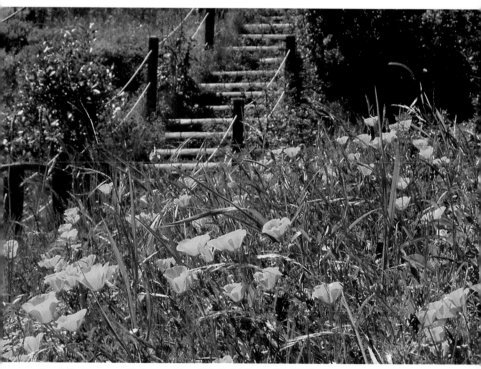

Presidio Nursery Stairway, Fort Winfield Scott (Walk 9) *Presidio*

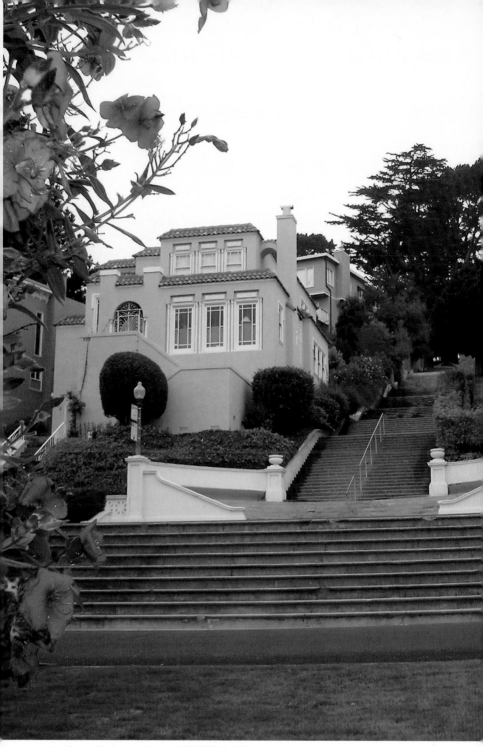

Pacheco Stairway, Forest Hill (Walk 15)

Tony Holiday

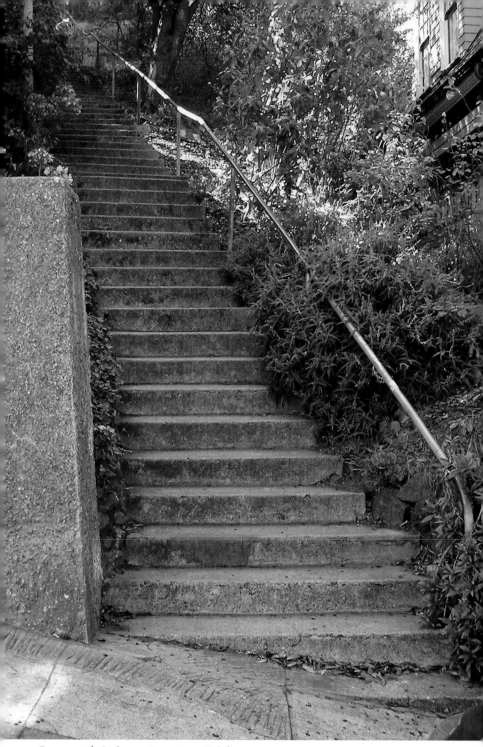

Farnsworth Stairway, Parnassus Heights *Tony Holiday*

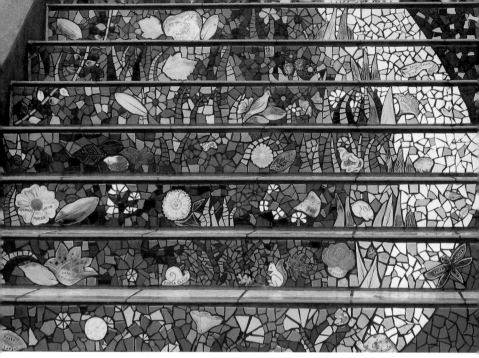

Mosaic tile stairway at 16th Ave. and Moraga (Walk 11)   *James Charney*

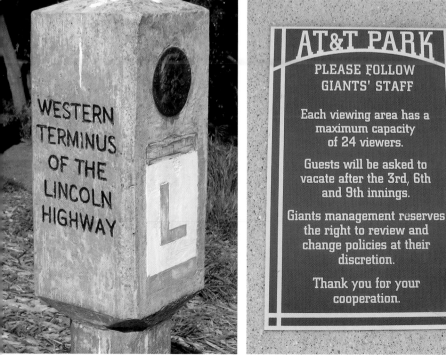

Lincoln memorial post (Walk 10)
Tony Holiday

WESTERN
TERMINUS
OF THE
LINCOLN
HIGHWAY

L

AT&T PARK

PLEASE FOLLOW GIANTS' STAFF

Each viewing area has a maximum capacity of 24 viewers.

Guests will be asked to vacate after the 3rd, 6th and 9th innings.

Giants management reserves the right to review and change policies at their discretion.

Thank you for your cooperation.

Free View **sign at AT&T Park (Walk 29)**
Tony

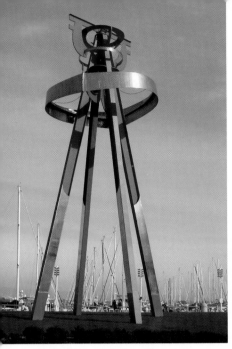

Mark di Suvero's *Sea Change* (Walk 29) *Tony Holiday*

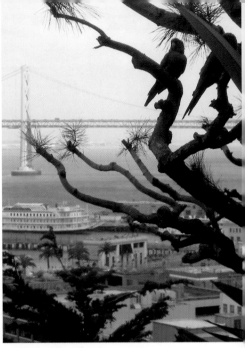

A view of the Bay from Calhoun Terrace (Walk 1) *James Charney*

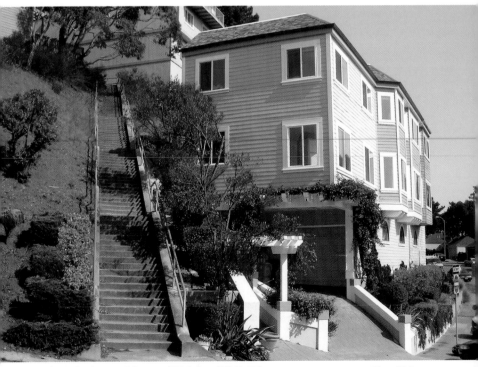

Onique Stairway, Diamond Heights (Walk 25) *Tony Holi-*

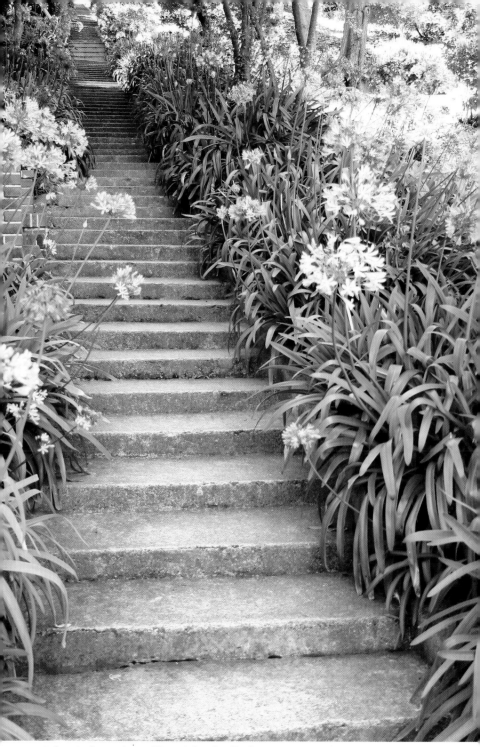

Baker Stairway in Pacific Heights (Walk 7) *Polly Gates*

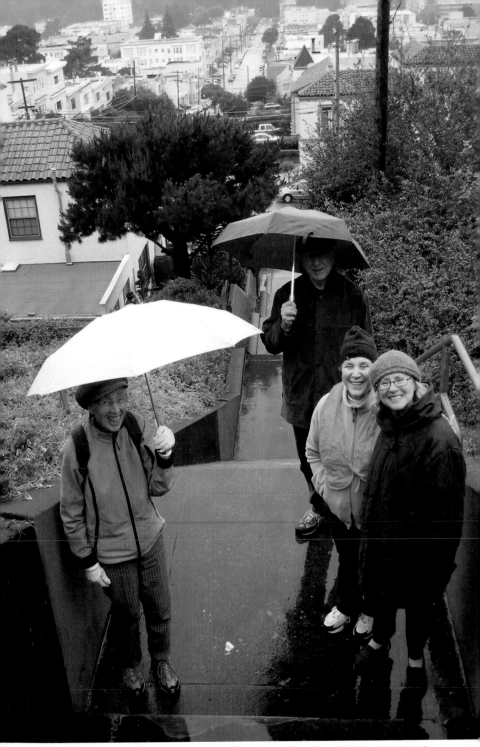

Adah Bakalinsky (left) and fellow walkers in Golden Gate Heights (Walk 11)
James Charney

Treasures

Yerba Buena Cove, Telegraph Hill, & Chinatown

& Digressions

The early Spanish explorers of the 18th century designated three important foci in the city: religious—Mission Dolores; military—The Presidio; and commercial—Yerba Buena Cove. In this walk we'll explore the commercial area.

You will see buildings that were erected on the edge of the shoreline along the middle third of Yerba Buena Cove, now the financial and commercial section of San Francisco. You walk toward Portsmouth Square, which was the center of the Pueblo of Yerba Buena and now is the center of Chinatown; you continue to the slopes of Telegraph Hill where the 19th-century waterfront workers lived. You may feel you are traveling through a land of plaques in Walks 1 and 2. The northeast part of the city is a small, concentrated area where the early Spanish commercial history of San Francisco began. The plaques are well-written and don't overburden you with a multitude of facts; they include just enough to stir up your imagination.

The Gold Rush to California was the Outward Bound of the 1800s, the 19th-century rite of passage. It took all of one's ingenuity, statesmanship, business acumen, and physical stamina to survive. San Francisco, the entry point for people coming overland by wagon and around the Horn by ship, had a population of approximately 450 at the first census count in 1847 and approximately 20,000 by the end of 1849. Gradually, as more families arrived in the city, social services were organized; schools, libraries, and churches were opened; lectures, operas, concerts, readings, and theater were offered.

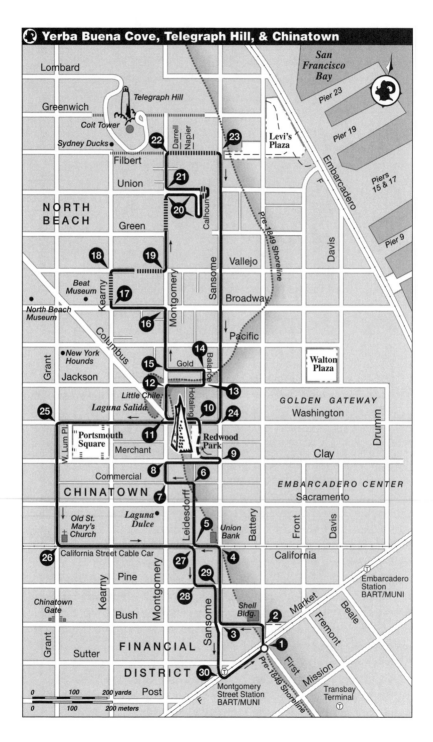

Lombard

Greenwich

Telegraph Hill

Coit Tower

Sydney Ducks

Filbert

Union

NORTH BEACH

Green

22

Darrell

Napier

23

Levi's Plaza

Pier 23

Pier 19

Piers 15 & 17

Pier 9

San Francisco Bay

Embarcadero

Davis

21

Calhoun

20

Pre-1849 Shoreline

18

19

Vallejo

Broadway

Pacific

17

Beat Museum

Kearny

North Beach Museum

Columbus

16

New York Hounds

Jackson

Grant

15

14

Gold

Balance

Montgomery

Sansome

12

Little Chile

Laguna Salida

13

Hotaling

10

24

Walton Plaza

GOLDEN GATEWAY
Washington

Drumm

25

11

Portsmouth Square

Merchant

Redwood Park

8

Commercial

6

9

Clay

EMBARCADERO CENTER
Sacramento

CHINATOWN

7

Old St. Mary's Church

Laguna Dulce

Leidesdorff

5

Union Bank

Battery

Front

Davis

26

California Street Cable Car

Pine

4

California

Embarcadero Station BART/MUNI

Chinatown Gate

Kearny

Montgomery

27

29

28

Sansome

Shell Bldg.

Market

Beale

Fremont

Bush

2

Grant

Sutter

FINANCIAL

3

1

First

Mission

DISTRICT

30

Post

Montgomery Street Station BART/MUNI

Pre-1849 Shoreline

Transbay Terminal

| 0 | 100 | 200 yards |
| 0 | 100 | 200 meters |

WALK 1 ROUTE: Yerba Buena Cove, Telegraph Hill, & Chinatown

Public Transportation: The many streetcars, buses, or Metro lines that run along Market are useful for reaching this route. For MUNI bus information, call 311 (outside San Francisco call (415) 701-2311).

1. Begin at 1st and Market. Cross Market to the intersection of Battery and Bush.
2. Left on Bush.
3. Right on Sansome to California. Cross to far side.
4. Left on California to Leidesdorff.
5. Right on Leidesdorff to Commercial.
6. Left on Commercial to Montgomery.
7. Right on Montgomery to Clay.
8. Right on Clay, a few yards past Redwood Park to Two Transamerica Center to see the Niantic plaque.
9. Return to walk through the park to Sansome. (The Washington St. gate is open during business hours from Monday to Friday. During this time, you can exit directly to Washington.)
10. Left on Washington to Montgomery.
11. Right on Montgomery to Jackson.
12. Right on Jackson to Balance.
13. Left on Balance to Gold.
14. Left on Gold to Montgomery.
15. Right (north) on Montgomery to Broadway.
16. Left on Broadway to Kearny.
17. Right to ascend Kearny Stwy. to Vallejo.
18. Right to descend Vallejo Stwy. to Montgomery.
19. Left to ascend Montgomery Stwy. to Union.
20. Right turn into Union cul-de-sac. Descend stairway on left to walkway. Ascend stairway on right to Calhoun Terrace and turn left.
21. Return to Montgomery and turn right to Filbert.
22. Right on Filbert to descend stairway to Sansome.
23. Right turn on Sansome to Washington.
24. Right on Washington to right side of Grant to see No. 823 (some merchandise belonging to the adjoining boutique may hide the number, but it's there).
25. Left (south) on Grant to California.
26. Left on California to Leidesdorff.
27. Right on Leidesdorff to Pine.
28. Left on Pine to Sansome.
29. Right on Sansome to Market.
30. Left on Market to 1st to your beginning.

Telegraph Hill, at 284 feet in elevation, extended east to Battery, near the edge of the Bay, making it difficult to unload cargo. After the east slope of the hill was quarried, it extended just to the west side of Sansome. Dock workers living in the small cottages along the hillside used a stairway to go to and from work. During the late 19th and early 20th centuries, artists, writers, and actors lived on the hill. Junius Booth of the famous theater family lived at No. 5 Calhoun Terrace. The writer, Charles Warren Stoddard, spent part of his childhood here at No. 287 Union. The hill became a special province due in part to its isolated site.

⬦ Begin at Market and 1st St. (the first street west of Yerba Buena Cove, now about a half mile from the Ferry Bldg. and the Bay). An interpretive plaque is embedded in the sidewalk. No. 525 Market, the Cushman-Wakefield Bldg., straddles the shoreline. During the week visitors can see the current art exhibits in the lobby.

⬦ Cross Market to the intersections of Battery, Bush, and Market. At the corner near the *Mechanics Monument* is another embedded plaque showing the map of Yerba Buena Cove. The *Mechanics Monument* was commissioned in 1894 by Peter Donahue to honor his father, James Donahue, founder of Union Iron Works. The foundry, one of the most successful firms in early San Francisco, was located on Harrison, which provided easy access to the Bay. Douglas Tilden, known as the Michelangelo of the West, sculpted the figures on the monument. Although he had been deaf since childhood, his talent was recognized early, and he was able to study in Paris.

⬦ Cross Battery at Bush to see another building that straddles the cove—the 29-story Shell Bldg. at 100 Bush. George Pelham designed and built it in 1929–1930. Consistent restoration work has preserved the Art Deco detailing. The shell motif is repeated in the transom, as a light fixture, and in the lobby. At night, the building is suffused with a golden light. Walk over to 130 Bush to see the Heineman Bldg., an anomaly and a curiosity. It is the narrowest building in San Francisco. Three steps into the lobby, and one is almost in the elevator.

⬦ Continue west to Sansome, and then north to California. The Union Bank straddles the shoreline at No. 400 California. It was originally the Bank of California, founded in 1864 by William Ralston and O. J. Mills. Bliss and Faville, famous for their classical government buildings, designed it in 1907–1908 in Beaux Arts style, beautiful and elegant, but everything is oversized, perfect for a display of power and wealth, and it makes me feel like a Lilliputian. (Two of their other buildings I am fond of are The Convent of the Sacred Heart School [1912] and the St. Francis Hotel [1904, rebuilt in 1907].) The 21-story tower incorporated into the bank structure was designed by Anshen and Allen in 1967. The integration of the old and new edifices is considered one of the most successful and aesthetic in the city, and the coffered ceiling is elegant. Two plaques near the entrance of the bank provide a fine introduction to a visit of the interior to which you are welcome. The historic exhibit downstairs has artifacts from the early days of gold mining, including a cabinet with pieces of gold that were exchanged for money. The museum is open Monday through Friday.

◢ Continue west (to your left) on California to the intersection of Leidesdorff, which marks the old shoreline. It is named for Captain William Alexander Leidesdorff, a prosperous businessman, linguist, and master of the ship *Julia Ann*, which carried Hawaiian sugar that was traded for California hides. Leidesdorff also was active in fur trading with the Russians at Fort Ross. He settled in Yerba Buena in 1838 and built the City Hotel at Kearny and Clay, and a warehouse on the beach at California and Leidesdorff. The captain, born of Danish and African ancestry in the Virgin Islands, died of cholera in 1848 at the age of 36.

◢ Walk to your right through Leidesdorff toward Sacramento. Read the plaque that details the history of What Cheer House (left side of the street), a hotel built by R. B. Woodward in 1852. He later added a private library and museum for guests, an unusual facility for hotels to offer. Captain Ulysses S. Grant stayed there in 1854. (Woodward's Gardens near Mission and 14th St. was the popular outdoor resort in the city in the 1860s.) Laguna Dulce, a freshwater pond fed by a Nob Hill stream, was situated a half block away at Montgomery and Sacramento. It was also the site of a Native American sweat lodge.

◢ Continue on Leidesdorff to Commercial St. (You are standing in water.) Turn left to Montgomery to stand in the place where Captain Montgomery sailed up in the USS *Portsmouth*, in 1846, to claim the Pueblo of Yerba Buena (established in 1839) for the United States. The Mexican government acceded. It was a quiet takeover. The Pacific Heritage Museum at 608 Commercial (free and open Thursday–Saturday, 10 AM–4 PM) has exhibits relating to Chinese history and customs.

◢ Continue on Montgomery to Clay. Read the plaque on the side of No. 550, at the southeast corner where the Bank of Italy was located in 1904. In the early years, the bank used solicitors to sell accounts. Across the street is the Transamerica Pyramid. The original building on this site was the 1853 Montgomery Block, affectionately known as the Monkey Block. Designed and built by architect Gordon Cummings for Henry Halleck, it was also known as Halleck's Folly because it cost $2 million. Four stories high, it had a fish market, grocery, and the Saloon Bank Exchange Bar, where bankers transacted business. In later years law offices and the largest law library in the area were located in the Monkey Block. Sun Yat-sen, founder of the Chinese Nationalist movement, had his office here during his exile, around 1911. In the 1920s and 1930s, artists, writers, and dancers rented studio and living quarters here. Among them were Pietro Mezzara—the sculptor, who made the first statue of Abraham Lincoln; George Sterling—the poet; and Ann Munstock, who brought modern dance to San Francisco from Germany.

◢ The Monkey Block withstood the 1906 earthquake but was torn down in 1954 to be used as a parking lot. The Transamerica Pyramid, built in 1972, superseded the parking lot. Its precarious site on the shoreline necessitated a 9-foot-thick concrete and steel foundation that extends 52 feet below the sidewalk. The building has become recognized as a San Francisco icon. I like the diminishing space it occupies as it continues upward. Since 9/11 the garage and interior areas beyond the lobby are closed to the general public.

◢ Continue right on Clay and walk past the Redwood Park (established by Transamerica for its employees and the public), to Two Transamerica Center to read the Niantic plaque. The Niantic Bldg. at No. 505 Sansome was named for the abandoned ship that provided one side of the structure. The crew left for the gold mines in 1849, and the vessel was converted into a hotel. (The plaque at the location where the ship was used as a warehouse is on the Clay side of 505 Sansome.) Artifacts from the ship found during excavation of the Transamerica Pyramid site are displayed on the 14th Floor of Washington Towers at No. 655 Montgomery (open Monday–Friday, 9 AM–5 PM).

◢ Return to and walk through Redwood Park, which is open Monday through Friday during business hours. It is a popular place for people to bring their lunch and, during the summer, listen to noon jazz concerts. It is also a sculpture garden and has two of my favorite outdoor pieces. The bronze *Puddle Jumpers* by Glenna Goodacre is a group of six children, whose movements—jumping rope, skipping, and hopping—are caught in mid-air and expressed with great joy and abandon. *The Frog Pond* by Richard Clopton is a group of brass frogs that exhibit the same delight in their pool.

◢ Exit the park on Washington. Turn left on Washington toward Montgomery. (On weekends go east on Clay to Sansome and then left to Washington). Cross Montgomery so that you can walk to your right on the odd-numbered side. Washington and Montgomery is a historic "corner." At the tip of it, No. 701, is the triangular "flatiron" structure built in 1911. (The Registered Landmark Plaque No. 52 is on the Columbus side near the entrance.) The building has undergone several metamorphoses—from the Fugazi Bank to the Bank of Italy to headquarters of Transamerica Corporation and currently, the Church of Scientology. Continue up Montgomery, and next to No. 735 is a plaque put in place by the California Centennials Commission and the Society of California Pioneers. The plaque refers to the New York Store, a two-story wood structure that was located here. As well as selling general merchandise, the store was the receiving, sorting, and dispersal point for the first regulation mail shipment that arrived on the steamer *Oregon* in 1849. The second historic event in the store was the celebration of the Jewish New Year in September 1849 by a group of 40 Jewish pioneers who used the second floor of the store as a synagogue. If you look up at the fire escape landings (one for each of the three floors), you will see three Stars of David on each railing that refer to this use.

◢ Continue on Montgomery to Jackson. The bridge that crossed Laguna Salida, the brackish inlet of the Yerba Buena Cove was located here. At No. 498, you pass the Lucas Turner & Co. Bank of 1853. General Sherman, famous for his march through Georgia during the Civil War, was director for several years. A historic plaque is on the wall.

◢ During the Gold Rush, Jackson and Montgomery was the center of Little Chile. Chilenos, expert at using the Chile wheel to crush gold-bearing ore, had come to work in the gold mines. (A plaque commemorating 7,000 Chilean miners is at Kearny and Columbus.) The Sydney Ducks—the Australian convict contingent—lived around the base of Telegraph Hill from Filbert, north, between

Montgomery and Kearny. The Hounds—a group of New York toughs—lived around Grant and Pacific. The latter two groups were "hate groups," intent on eradicating people from Central and South America. Finally, after a particularly vengeful foray into Little Chile, the Vigilante group of 1851 (who called themselves the Law and Order Party) was formed under Sam Brannan's leadership to combat the plundering and marauding by the Hounds and Ducks.

⚐ You are in the Jackson Square Historic District, which encompasses the area from Washington to Pacific and from Columbus to Sansome. The buildings in the 400 block of Jackson withstood the earthquake and fire of 1906, and the street has many of the earliest structures in San Francisco. Continue to the right on Jackson to Balance, the shortest street in the City. As you pass Hotaling Alley, look up at the Transamerica Pyramid. The alley was named for A. P. Hotaling's famed saloon and distillery (No. 429 Jackson). The famous two-line verse that was quoted after the quake posed a question: "If as they say God spanked the town for being over frisky / Why did he burn the churches down and save Hotaling's whiskey?"

⚐ Turn left on Balance (named for the sunken ship that lies at Jackson and Front) to Gold, one of the numerous alleys in this part of the City. The old three-story brick buildings are still here. (On the left is the side door of Stout Books.) Turn left on Gold to Montgomery, and then right (north) toward Broadway. During the winter of 1849–1850, 50 inches of rain was reported. Montgomery, unpaved and unplanked, was a treacherous thoroughfare, especially at night. Wagons sank into the mud, and inebriated pedestrians had to be pulled out. An unforgettable event of that winter was the discovery of three men's bodies in the mud along Montgomery.

⚐ William Stout Architectural Books at No. 804 Montgomery has one of the most complete selections in the country of books about and relating to architecture. I love to browse here. Japanesque Gallery at No. 824 Montgomery is my favorite stop for an aesthetic experience.

⚐ Pacific Ave. interests me because it illustrates so many contrasts in a few blocks. To our left where No. 549 Pacific stands (at Kearny), the scapula of a mammoth was dug up. (Hundreds of thousands of years ago mammoths and bison roamed around here in a wet area that resembled southern Marin County.) To our right, the street is lined on both sides, predominantly with ficus trees. Behind the trees, the 19th-century, three-story brick structures contrast greatly in size with the enormous pyramid and the Bank of California. The old structures have the ambiance of a small town where you could call out the first names of all the inhabitants. At the same time, during the Gold Rush days, the section of Pacific closer to Sansome was the notorious Barbary Coast, where gangs and crime were rampant.

⊿ Continue to Broadway. At the corner of Montgomery is the On Lok organization's Senior Health Services Center, which includes 35 apartments for low-income elderly. Seniors are brought by van and stay for the day to receive health and personal care and the midday meal. They participate in social and recreation activities and return home in the evening. One of the exciting programs is the ongoing, intergenerational garden shared by the frail elderly and about 24 children, ages two to five, from the Child Care program. The garden, transformed from an abandoned cement playground by the San Francisco League of Urban Gardeners, was additionally funded by several groups, among them, San Francisco Beautiful.

⊿ Turn left on Broadway to Kearny. As you ascend, you see remains of the earlier cobblestone paving underneath your feet. Turn right to ascend the sidewalk stairway to Vallejo. At eye level you have a view of the green flatiron Zoetrope Bldg. and the pedestrian bridge from the Hilton Hotel to Portsmouth Square.

⊿ Turn right on Vallejo. As you walk east, you come to the house at No. 448-B Vallejo. It was here that Madame Luisa Tetrazzini (1871–1940), the famous Italian opera soprano, while out walking (she was on tour in San Francisco) heard the young—12 or 13 years of age—Lina Pagliughi (born 1907), singing. Tetrazzini told Lina's parents she wanted to take their daughter to Italy to teach her opera and help launch her career as the second Madame Tetrazzini. The parents refused, but four years later, Lina did travel to Italy to begin her vocal studies under the direction of Tetrazzini. She subsequently had a long career with the Metropolitan Opera.

⊿ Walk down the Vallejo Stairway, designed by the Department of Public Works. The Department of Urban Forestry planted the trees and shrubs and maintains them. Neighbors have taken responsibility for additional plantings. Several years ago I spoke with residents in their 70s and 80s who lived adjacent to the stairway. They attributed their longevity to daily stairway walking.

◢ Turn left on Montgomery, walk past the three ginko trees, and ascend the stairway to Union. Look back to see Montgomery where it ends at Market. On a sunny day, you see Montgomery in shadow because of the high-rise buildings.

◢ Turn right into the Union cul-de-sac. No. 291 Union is the oldest house on that block, dating from 1861. The high retaining wall that separates Calhoun Terrace was built by the Works Progress Administration in 1939. Turn right into upper Calhoun Terrace. No. 9 Calhoun was built in 1854. Because it had its own spring, the owners did not request connection to the City water system until 1872. Walk back to Union and turn right into lower Calhoun Terrace. No. 66 built in 1939 was designed by a Viennese architect, Richard Neutra, who espoused the International Style.

◢ At the corner of Calhoun Terrace and Union descend the stairway. Looking down you will experience your elevation to Sansome St. (about 250 feet). There is no stairway down to the street because of the hazardous cliff conditions. Impatiens, century plants, snap-dragons, bottlebrush, and fuchsia dot the cliff. At this site, you will likely have a good view of the wild parrots of Telegraph Hill in the cypress trees, perching and preening and teasing each other. Their cocktail hour seems to be between 4 and 5 PM.

> *"If you stand around and look, you can see a lot."*
>
> —Yogi Berra

◢ Ascend the stairway on the left to Union. Nos. 287, 291, and 291-A were built in the 1860s. Return to Montgomery, turn right and stop for a moment in the middle of the street to look at No. 1360. The exterior is in the shape of a ship, complete with a shiplike upper deck. Etched into the glass over the central entrance are a gazelle, palm trees, and ocean waves. The etched panels on the side of the Art Moderne apartment house show The Worker holding the world above the Bay Bridge. The real 1937 Bay Bridge Towers are just beyond it. No. 1360 is also famous as the setting for the 1947 movie *Dark Passage*, which stars Humphrey Bogart and Lauren Bacall.

◢ On your left along the retaining wall is a well-designed garden and a humorous mural featuring an apricot-colored teacup poodle named Ginger. Dick Fosselman and Rick Helf, the artists, cleverly incorporated the actual water hydrant into the scene. The garden and the mural compose yet another of the surprisingly beautiful spots in the neighborhoods. From here, before descending the historic Filbert Stairway on the left side of No. 1360, a more complete view of the etched murals is available.

 A plaque on the Filbert Stairway expresses appreciation of Grace Marchant, who moved to the Filbert Stairway in 1950, when the area was a dumping ground 30 feet deep. The city permitted her to burn the dump; it took three days to burn completely. For 30 years Marchant labored on the stairway gardens, which were dedicated to her on May 4, 1980. She died in 1982 at the age of 96. Her neighbor, friend, and protégé, Gary Kray, cares for the gardens, and the city contributes water for their maintenance.

 Darrell Place and Napier Lane are "paper streets." Although they appear as streets on maps and in street guides, Darrell is more like a trail, while Napier consists only of 12-foot wood planks. Filbert is a wood stairway threading alongside the garden. Because fire is always a hazard in these areas where there is no room for trucks, the Fire Department stores equipment as inconspicuously as possible. Next to the blue fire hydrants on the walkway (blue is the code for connection to a high-pressure system) is a storage box for two small fire hydrants and a hose. The Gothic cottage at No. 228 (1873) was once a grocery. Next door, No. 226 is a renovated miner's shack from 1863.

Filbert Stairway *Tony Holiday*

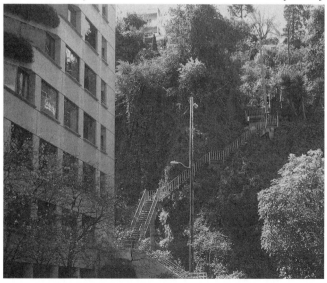

- The lower part of Filbert Stairway is concrete. Much of the overgrowth of nasturtiums, fennel, and blackberries growing along the sides of the hill has been cut down. The design of the patterned aggregate Levi's Plaza across the street pulls us forward as we descend to Sansome. The landscaping by Lawrence Halprin Associates includes granite and trees to evoke the Sierra, where Levi Strauss began his career in 1851. Strauss supplied miners with heavy duck cloth pants, reinforced with copper rivets, to withstand the pulling and the tearing from tools. The cloth was *serge de Nîmes* (from Nîmes, in southern France)—hence, denim. If the Levi Strauss Museum is open, walk in and look around.

- Cross Sansome and turn right to walk on the sidewalk. As we stroll, we become aware of the craggy east slope of Telegraph Hill, the result of years of unprofessional and unsupervised quarrying by the Gray Bros. (1890–1903). A women's group led by Alice Griffith and Elizabeth Ashe (founders of the Telegraph Hill Neighborhood Association) enlisted support from women citywide, to save Telegraph Hill from further damage. Momentum gathered, City Hall heard, and the Gray Bros.' permit was revoked.

- The extraordinary plantings here now are the efforts of two neighbors who rappelled down the hill to do the work. In spring, the hillside near Green is ablaze with color from Mexican sage, primroses, poppies, dudleya, valerian, morning glory, tree dahlias, potato vine and passion vine. Echium grows at the edge of the hill along the street. A plaque at No. 202 Green is dedicated to Philo Farnsworth who had his laboratory there from 1926 to 1938 when he was perfecting the first functional television system. He filed more than 80 television patents.

- Cross Sansome to the south corner of Green for an extraordinary view up the cliff. The backsides of three Calhoun Terrace houses supported by stilts are visible. They look as though they are imminently ready to inch forward toward Sansome.

- Continue on Sansome to Broadway. Cross to One Jackson Place between Pacific and Jackson. It is a breezeway (open Monday–Friday, 8 AM–6 PM) with businesses that extend to Battery. Then walk to the corner of Battery and Jackson to get a feeling of the water geography of the mid-1800s in the City. You are now, figuratively, standing in water deep enough to have the ship *Arkansas* dock here. The Old Ship Restaurant is at the location of that sunken ship where sailors were shanghaied. A plaque outside the restaurant has the history of the saloon. Walk on Jackson to see the name of the proprietor of that time, Henry Klee, on the top of the building. Walk back to Sansome and continue to Washington.

- Turn right on Washington to Grant. At Kearny we see Portsmouth Square, the heart and outdoor living room of Chinatown, formerly the center of the Pueblo of Yerba Buena. You are dipping a toe into Chinatown, a densely populated 25-block area. It was destroyed in the 1906 earthquake but rebuilt within two years. Many of the ornate buildings were decorated in the 1920s when a concerted effort was made by the community to attract visitors. Grant is the tourist shopping avenue. Stockton is where the Chinese residents and knowledgeable shoppers from neighboring areas come to buy fresh produce and oriental foods at the most reasonable prices. On the right side of Grant, at No. 823, is a plaque commemorating the first tent dwelling in Yerba Buena, which was erected in June 1835 by William Richardson, an Englishman who had deserted the English whaler *Orion* 13 years before. Industrious and helpful to the community, Richardson married the commandant's daughter and became a naturalized citizen. The plaque is on the wall on the right side of the door. The display of merchandise from the adjoining store partially covered it when I was there, but I gently brushed them aside to reveal it. (There were many hotels and theaters in this area during the 1850s—the Jenny Lind, the Phoenix, the Adelphi, the Italian Theater, and some better-known Chinese theaters.)

- Turn left on Grant to California. At the northeast corner is Old St. Mary's, the first Catholic cathedral in San Francisco, dedicated in 1854. It was rebuilt after being damaged in the 1906 earthquake. Still an active parish, Old St. Mary's presents a fine noon concert series and an outreach program. You turn left on California, right on Leidesdorff, and then left on Pine. Walking toward Sansome, you can see the 1930 Pacific Exchange at No. 301 Pine (now the Equinox Fitness Center) and the Ralph Stackpole sculpture that reflects the massiveness of the building designed primarily by Timothy Pfleuger, of Miller and Pfleuger, architects. He was famous for the large theaters he built—the Castro and Alhambra in the City and the Paramount in Oakland. One of my favorite clocks in the City is on the Furth Bldg. at the northwest corner of Sansome. It is flanked by a lion on the left and a unicorn on the right.

- Turn right on Sansome to Market, and then turn left on Market to 1st St. to your beginning.

Further Ambling

To experience the water beneath you, walk over what once was Yerba Buena Cove. Start your walk at Commercial and Sansome in the courtyard that leads to the Embarcadero Buildings walkway. Pass the sculpture and fountain to the stairways and ascend either one. Continue on the walkway along the One, Two, Three, and Four Embarcadero Buildings. You will descend at the Embarcadero.

Old

Telegraph Hill & North Beach

Neighborhoods

You begin the walk in a historic area of North Beach—at the intersection of Mason and Bay. During the Gold Rush days, North Beach extended only to Francisco St., near the water line. Henry "Honest Harry" Meiggs, a New York State lumberman, built a sawmill and one of the first wharfs extending into the Bay (between Mason and Powell) and established a thriving lumber trade (with imports from Oregon). Genial, well liked, and a cofounder of the San Francisco Philharmonic Society, he knew politicians and power brokers and invested heavily in real estate in North Beach and neighborhoods farther west, believing that the area would develop rapidly. He was wrong. Meiggs found himself in the untenable position of being personally bankrupt, and, since he had embezzled City funds, responsible for a financial crisis in San Francisco. Banks closed, many permanently, and investors lost their savings. In 1854, "Honest Harry" managed to sail away to Chile, where he subsequently made another fortune building a railroad through the mountains to Peru. Though he repaid most of his San Francisco debts, he died in Lima in 1877, having been denied return to California.

During the 1850s, the North Beach waterfront was a dynamic community. Conditions were in flux: there were so many people coming in, both from the eastern U.S. and overseas. Some were in transit, but others came to settle here. Supportive services were established—fishing boats, breweries, forges, and slaughterhouses; there were restaurants, saloons, import stores, and hostelries.

The 1906 earthquake leveled everything in this quarter except the Ferry Bldg., which at that time was the tallest structure in San Francisco. The area was soon rebuilt, and the City celebrated its rebirth with the Panama-Pacific International Exposition of 1915.

Over the years the San Francisco port has diminished in importance. The thrust of the Port Authority's master plan is to balance maritime needs and the needs of the public. One of the plans for Fisherman's Wharf is to centralize the fish wholesalers in one facility, and return the area to its original purpose—catching, preparing, and selling fish to residents and tourists alike.

Along the Embarcadero, the Pier 7 Esplanade is a popular site for walking, fishing, and picnicking; Piers 80–96 are the container terminals.

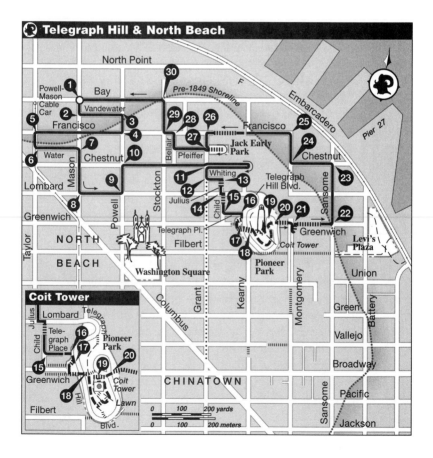

WALK 2 ROUTE: Telegraph Hill & North Beach

Public Transportation: Cable car; MUNI Bus #39 Coit; #30 Stockton. For MUNI bus information, call 311 (outside San Francisco call (415) 701-2311).

1. Begin at Mason and Bay. Walk south on Mason to Vandewater.
2. Left on Vandewater to Powell.
3. Right on Powell to Francisco.
4. Right on Francisco to Taylor.
5. Left on Taylor to Water.
6. Left on Water to Mason.
7. Right on Mason to Lombard.
8. Left on Lombard to Powell.
9. Left on Powell to Chestnut.
10. Right on Chestnut past Grant to end of street. Return to Grant.
11. Left to No. 1834 Grant at Whiting.
12. Left on Whiting.
13. Midway on right, ascend Julius St. Stwy. and walkway to Lombard.
14. Left to No. 383 Lombard and ascend Child St. Stwy. and walkway to Telegraph Place.
15. Left on Telegraph Place to Telegraph Hill Blvd.
16. Keep right and continue up Telegraph Hill Blvd.
17. Two doors from No. 201, descend stairway into Greenwich cul-de-sac. Walk around planted area; ascend stairway to Telegraph Hill Blvd.
18. Cross Blvd. to ascend stone stairway. Cross path to new donor stairways and ascend to front of Coit Tower and JCDecaux toilet area.
19. Walk to the plaque designed by Michael Manwaring below stairway in front of tower. Explore area and then continue on paths around tower.
20. Go around to the front of the Tower, then bear right to cross the boulevard and descend the Greenwich Stwy. to Montgomery.
21. Cross Montgomery. Go right to lower Montgomery. Next to No. 1460, descend to continue down Greenwich Stwy.
22. Left on Sansome to Chestnut.
23. Left on Chestnut to Montgomery.
24. Right on Montgomery to Francisco.
25. Left on Francisco. Ascend stairway to Francisco cul-de-sac and Grant.
26. Left on Grant to ascend stairway to Jack Early Park on left side of street.
27. Return to Grant and cross the street to walk through Pfeiffer St. to Bellair Place to Francisco.
28. Left on Francisco to Stockton.
29. Right on Stockton to Bay.
30. Left on Bay to Mason to your beginning.

- From the intersection of Mason and Bay, walk south on Mason. Turn left on Vandewater St. It was under water in 1849 and then in later years it evolved into a charming "twitton" as the British call it. The paved street is softened by trees and three- and four-story apartment buildings.

- Continue to Powell, and turn right on Francisco. The historical site at Nos. 411–445, until 1980, was the Bauer-Schweitzer Malt Company, the last barrel-malting factory west of the Mississippi. Their high-quality malt was sold to small American breweries such as Anchor, and was also exported to Japan. When it became economically unfeasible to continue operations, the building was sold. The North Beach Malt House condominium complex is an exemplary historic conversion. During construction I was able to see the interior, and I was impressed with the imaginative use of malting equipment in sculptures designed for the courtyard, and the placement of historical displays in the lobbies. It is not open to the public.

- Turn left onto Taylor and then turn left again onto Water, another block-long twitton. It is a remnant of early San Francisco fish houses, warehouses, and bordellos. Turn right on Mason.

- Continue on Mason to No. 661 Lombard to view the renovated Joe DiMaggio North Beach Playground and pool. No. 660 Lombard, the Telegraph Hill Neighborhood Center, was founded in 1890 by Elizabeth Ashe and Alice Griffith to provide services to low-income immigrant families. Their efforts focused on resisting the quarrying of the hill, providing a settlement house at the crest of Vallejo for nursing care, a boys' club, and classes in homemaking and family counseling. When the newcomers realized these services were genuine, they began giving fruit and vegetables to the house, and an evening club for girls working in the canneries was begun. Griffith and Ashe were inspired by the work of Jane Addams of Chicago's Hull House, and that spirit continues today.

- After the 1906 earthquake they set up a tent city in Washington Square Park and worked on legislation to prevent sleazy rebuilding. Currently, the program at the neighborhood center includes health and educational services to new immigrants from the Pacific Rim, to seniors, and to children from preschool age and older. Gardening is a favorite activity for all generations at the center, as evidenced by the inviting flower beds in the front and vegetable garden in the back.

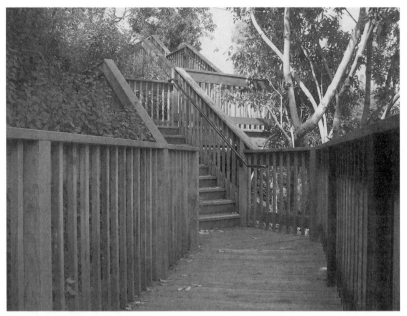

Francisco Stairway *Tony Holiday*

◢ One of the most abundant displays of cascading, fuchsia-colored bougainvillea in the City adorns No. 604 Lombard. The vine was planted in 1938; it blooms twice a year, and each year it becomes more exuberant. The contrast of its color with the six junipers (their shapes suggest ladybugs) planted along the wall of the apartment house is an additional reward.

◢ Turn left on Powell and right on Chestnut. Continue walking two blocks to Grant and Chestnut. No. 298 Chestnut is a Mediterranean-style home built in 1929. Its tile roof, marble entry, and ceramic Della Robbia plaque are visible through the iron gates. Walk to the end of the Kearny cul-de-sac along the left side (designated as "open space") to obtain a view of the "lowlands." Here you have a long view of Marin County toward the north and west. Besides the boats anchored at Pier 39, you can see Piers 35 and 33 and perhaps a container ship proceeding toward the Port of Oakland. Pier 39 is well-known for its fine horticultural displays of container-flowers, the colony of sea lions that have taken up residence along the wharf, the good restaurants, and friendly stores. The outdoor spaces encourage strolling, and the area is very popular with young people and children. It's a great place to

Telegraph Hill & North Beach 23

watch fireworks on the Fourth of July. (These are important enough reasons to lessen my negative reaction to the architecture.) Angel Island State Park is to the north.

⊿ Return to Grant. At Grant turn left (south) and left again into Whiting cul-de-sac. Three-fourths of the way down the block and to the right, ascend the nine steps of Julius St. Stairway and walk to the end, which brings you to Lombard. Across the street to the left of No. 383 is the short Child St. Stairway.

⊿ Walk up to Telegraph Place and continue to Telegraph Hill Blvd. Turn right. Next to No. 201, descend a stairway into the Greenwich St. cul-de-sac. Circle around the planted oval area dedicated to Maria Pimentell for her 25 years of gardening. Walk up the opposite stairway to Telegraph Hill Blvd.

⊿ Cross the boulevard to ascend the stone stairway leading to the footpath. Cross the footpath and ascend the stairway with donors' names to the top. In the early days it was known as Signal Hill because the arrival of ships would be signaled from here across the City. In the 1880s, a restaurant was the chief attraction on the hill.

⊿ At the top, walk to the wall plaque designed by Michael Manwaring. It notates the historical timetable of the Pioneer Park Project. Arthur Brown, Jr.'s original landscape plan for the area surrounding the 1933 Coit Tower which he also designed, was finally completed in 2002! Fulfilling a historic mission to bring beauty to the park for all to share, it also emphasized contemporary history by inscribing on the stairs the names of people who contributed to the fund-raising. The Pioneer Park Project began as a dedicated, determined, and formidable pro bono grassroots group of volunteers who worked for six years to raise the money for the construction of three new stairways leading to Coit Tower, a picnic area overlooking the Bay, a wheelchair-accessible ramp, and the planting of native plants and trees. This large-scale beautification undertaking is one of the finest examples of commitment, intelligent planning, and consistent involvement by Telegraph Hill neighbors, as well as the cooperation of the City of San Francisco and other interested residents. The project matches in scale the 1876 purchase of the four lots at the crest of Telegraph Hill by San Francisco citizens, who subsequently transferred ownership to the City.

⊿ Coit Tower, dedicated in 1933, was funded by Lillie Hitchcock Coit, who had fond memories from childhood when she was a mascot for Knickerbocker Engine Company No. 5, one of the City's volunteer firefighting companies. The tower rises 179 feet from the crest of Telegraph Hill, itself 284 feet high.

⬛ Walk to the footpath on your right, where you will see an excellent map of San Francisco on the side of the JCDecaux public toilet. Continue to Pioneer Park, at the back of Coit Tower. There are low retaining walls where you can sit, have your lunch, and enjoy the views of eastern, southern, and western San Francisco. On a sunny day, everybody comes to Coit Tower to eat his or her lunch, enjoy the conviviality, and return to work refreshed.

⬛ The view to the east of the graceful 1895 Ferry Bldg. and its famous clock is distinctive. (Lit up at night, it is a cameo, a Cinderella, surpassing all other commercial buildings in its delicate beauty.)

⬛ The tall, slender Embarcadero buildings to the southeast are on the site of the old wholesale produce market. Because Embarcadero Center is on redevelopment land and federal funds partially defrayed building costs, the developer was obliged to spend one percent of the total project cost on art works. The result has been excellent sculpture located throughout the center. Directly in front of you is the Transamerica Pyramid, built on the original shoreline (Walk 1). The 48-story dark carnelian granite structure is the Bank of America Building on California.

⬛ As you walk along the right side of Coit Tower, look inside and see the Works Progress Administration murals executed in the 1930s. Intermittent vandalism and/or damage from water seepage have necessitated closing the mural rooms to visitors from time to time. The elevator ride to the top floor is available to the public at a nominal charge. The parking lot has coin telescopes to bring Marin County and the East Bay into close-up view.

⬛ Walk down the front stairs of the tower, take the footpath to the right, and cross Telegraph Hill Blvd. to descend the Greenwich Stairway. The upper brick section of the stairway curves, allowing room on each side for wide, terraced, private gardens. The unnamed lane running at a right angle from No. 356 Greenwich connects with the Filbert Stairway farther south (Walk 1).

⬛ The first landing of these 147 stairs leads down to the Montgomery cul-de-sac and the now closed Landmark 121 Julius Castle restaurant, built in 1923. A beautiful, mature fig tree graces the entrance. Because the lower retaining wall was designed in a random pattern of brick with protruding stones, which is extremely photogenic, I always look back before descending the next set of stairs.

- Cross Montgomery (you may feel like an opera singer taking a deep breath) and bear right to the Greenwich sign. Descend the concrete stairs and extended walkways. Along the way you see a cistern for firefighting, and, on the left side of the walkway, trees (a magnificent magnolia) and gardens (roses and irises, as well as ferns and fuchsias). The resident flock of wild parrots hangs out here and obtains sustenance from juniper berries and loquats near No. 243 Greenwich.

- Mark Bittner, who lives nearby, was able to watch the parrots from a vantage point where he did not frighten them. He observed them over a period of years, and they learned to trust him, eat from his

Telegraph Hill, ca. 1880

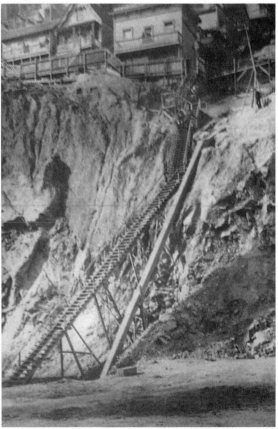

hand, and sit on his shoulder. When he began observing and feeding them, there were 25 in the flock. He says there are between 180 and 200 birds living on the hill. Mark learned their behavior patterns and their individual quirks, named them, and fed the flock for several years. He no longer feeds them because he says the parrots are finding enough food to eat on their own. They have been seen in Glen Park, Fort Mason, and Russian Hill, and they roost in Walton Square. The highly acclaimed documentary film *The Wild Parrots of Telegraph Hill* by Judy Irving has been seen throughout the United States and Europe. I like it very much, and also enjoyed Mark's book, a beautifully told story about how his life has been affected by the parrots, by Judy, and by his writing. In June 2006, Mark and Judy were married, and Telegraph Hill celebrated.

◢ The Parks, Trees, and Birds Committee of the Telegraph Hill Dwellers, under the leadership of Judy Irving, has taken on the responsibility of clearing overgrowth and invasive plants in the area. Hired professional arborists are removing dead wood and pruning the healthy trees. In clearing out and cutting back the ivy, they discovered a California coast live oak. It has several trunks and is probably 50 to 60 years old. There are fifteen varieties of trees in the canyon. Valetta Hazlett, daughter of Grace Marchant (Walk 1), planted the Deodar cedars 60 years ago. Along the footpath of the canyon, resident artists have randomly placed pieces of sculpture and mosaics and whimsical items, like the parking meter in back of the comfortable bench. These constantly change, but what a delight for residents and visitors to be alerted to these favors. The day I was there, I was surrounded by hummingbirds. At the foot of the steps, turn left on Sansome and continue north.

◢ The slope of Telegraph Hill, now barely visible from Sansome and Lombard since the Lombard Plaza apartments were built in 1991, was the amphitheater for a 1966 Janis Joplin rock concert.

◢ Turn left on Chestnut. A three-story brick structure (originally built in the late 1800s and reconstructed in 1973) is angled across the corner of Montgomery. You turn right on Montgomery and left on Francisco.

◢ At the cross street of Kearny, walk into the well-cared-for courtyard of the Wharf Plaza, a subsidized housing complex for seniors and families. The gardens are a pleasant place for the residents to sit and visit, and in September the area is spectacular with gingko trees ringed in gold leaves. Ascend the well-designed stairway. It features an unusual, long, elevated walkway—perfect for a stairway dance performance. At the top of the stairway you reach the Francisco cul-de-sac. The Telegraph Terrace condos fit snugly into the block and around the corner onto Grant.

◢ Turn left on Grant. In the middle of the block, make another left to walk up the stairs to Jack Early Park. Beginning in 1962 Jack Early ("Mr. Tree"), in a one-man effort, started planting trees and flowers in a neglected area. When I spoke to him, he remembered carrying water buckets by hand from his house on Pfeiffer. Now maintained by the Telegraph Terrace Association, the park is a rewarding place for views, solitude, and moon-watching.

◢ Come back down the stairway, cross Grant, and walk through Pfeiffer Alley, a right-of-way that has become a special enclave. Nos. 139–141 date from 1910, and No. 152 from 1891.

◢ Turn right into Bellair Place. Paving stones and recessed spaces for plants are welcoming tokens of promise. Make a left on Francisco and cross the street to see the little cottage at No. 276, which dates from 1863. Delicious aromas emanate from No. 271, Tante Marie's Cooking School.

◢ Continue west on Francisco to Stockton. Turn right to Bay, and left to the beginning of the walk.

◢ You have explored some of the alleyways and lanes and right-of-ways that are plentiful in North Beach. If you want to explore the neighborhood shopping areas on Columbus or upper Grant, you will find lots of foot traffic, small shops, restaurants, and coffeehouses with outdoor tables and chairs. Many of the old Italian businesses have closed; Chinese signs are common on stores.

◢ Those who have lived in the City for years are nostalgic about the old North Beach. Columbus Day (in fall) and the Blessing of the Fishing Fleet (in spring) were first celebrated in North Beach. Small opera houses on Green, Stockton, and Columbus were very well attended. At one time only Italian vaudeville was performed at the Flag Street Theater at Stockton and Columbus. Tom Cara introduced the espresso machine to the area from Italy after World War II.

◢ Enrico Banducci introduced new entertainers at his hungry i club (for "hungry intellectual"), including Barbra Streisand, Woody Allen, and the Kingston Trio. Comedians Lenny Bruce and Phyllis Diller first appeared at the Purple Onion, another comedy club also on Columbus. At one time 12 accordion makers were doing a lively business in North Beach. (In 1990 the Court of Historical

Review decided that the accordion was the official instrument of San Francisco.) The Beat poets held readings in the coffeehouses on upper Grant during the 1950s; Lawrence Ferlinghetti's City Lights bookstore still continues from those days (No. 261 Columbus). The zany revue *Beach Blanket Babylon* has been performed continuously since 1974.

Phyllis Pearsall (1906–1996), the founder of Geographer's A–Z Map Company, walked for 18 hours (beginning at 5 AM) daily, to list a total of 23,000 roads in London. Asked if she got lost in London, she replied, "Always, dear." During her lifetime, she walked 3,000 miles.

◢ Washington Square, the piazza on Stockton between Union and Filbert (now City Landmark No. 226), was reserved as a park in the City plan of 1847 and was one of the parks that sheltered the 1906 earthquake homeless in prefabricated camp cottages. Fragments of memories that people have shared over the years compose the ambiance of North Beach. First-time visitors will not share this background, but the abundance of specialty stores at street level, the number of eating places, the general friendliness, and the density of neighborhood foot traffic invite further exploring.

Further Ambling

If you'd like to shop for food or sundry items, you have choices available in all directions, within comfortable walking distance. You could walk south on Grant into the upper Grant area and Columbus. Many Asian restaurants plus the poultry, fish, and vegetable markets of Chinatown are one block west, on Stockton. The Cost Plus import store at No. 2552 Taylor is a popular place to buy inexpensive, imported trinkets, foods, and housewares. The Cannery, six blocks west at the foot of Columbus, at No. 2801 Leavenworth, is an unusual facility that offers shopping and the San Francisco Maritime National Historical Visitor Center (Walk 6). Ghirardelli Square (Walk 6), 900 North Point, two blocks beyond, another historic setting, has been converted to a residential/specialty shopping/dining complex.

Castles

Nob Hill

in the Air

Nob Hill, 376 feet above the Bay, is wedged between Pacific Heights to the west, Russian Hill to the north, and North Beach and Chinatown to the east. Millions of tourists have traversed Nob Hill on the cable cars, gliding both north-south on Powell between Market and Fisherman's Wharf, and east-west on California. The Powell line began operations in 1887; the California St. cable railway began in 1878.

A paradox of this walk is that the most interesting characteristics can be noted by standing still—looking up to make out the lofty architectural details on the buildings and registering at eye level the delight of cable car riders. Binoculars add extended range to your sightings.

Nob Hill is famous for its views, luxury hotels, and apartment houses. The only "neighbors" in this section may be doormen, hotel guests alighting from a taxi, or the elderly rich assisted by nurses or companions. But there is a neighborhood, and in the side streets and alleyways there are neighbors to visit and talk to, and who might even share garden cuttings. The Nob Hill Association, the neighborhood watchdog organization founded in 1923, is actively concerned with the environment and community issues.

The Donaldina Cameron House at No. 920 Sacramento was formerly the Chinese Presbyterian Mission Home. The mission began efforts in 1874 to rescue young Chinese girls brought to San Francisco as factory slaves and prostitutes. Donaldina Cameron joined the group in 1895 and continued her missionary work for 40 years. The house currently provides community recreational and social services. The clinker-brick structure was built in 1881 and then rebuilt in 1907 by Julia Morgan.

- ◢ You begin the walk at California and Leavenworth on the crest of Nob Hill. Walk north on Leavenworth, along the odd-numbered side for a few yards, and turn left into Acorn Alley. Usually it is full of plants and color during the growing season.

- ◢ From Acorn, turn left on Leavenworth toward Sacramento. Dashiell Hammett lived in the brick and stucco building on the corner at No. 1155 while he finished writing *The Maltese Falcon*. I always look for legends in a neighborhood. Chicos grocery store at No. 1168 Leavenworth was one when it was in the Chicos family from 1929 to 1997. (No longer owned by the family, it is still run as a grocery store with the same name.) Any long-time Nob Hill resident can tell you tales of the special favors the two brothers, then later their sons (cousins) did for their customers. Their grocery was a Nob Hill institution. When neighbors went on vacation, they left their keys with Chicos. Chicos always had access to their apartments to deliver groceries. When customers ordered items Chicos did not stock, the grocers secured it elsewhere. In emergencies, they used their truck to drive someone to the hospital or doctor.

- ◢ Cross Sacramento to see the corner building with two addresses, Nos. 1202–1206 Leavenworth and Nos. 1380–1390 Sacramento. Designed by Julia Morgan in 1910, it is a Craftsman-style shingle structure. Morgan worked in the San Francisco Bay Area from about 1905 to the 1930s, designing Craftsman-style homes and also elegant structures such as the Hearst Castle in San Simeon, California.

- ◢ Continue on Leavenworth to No. 1263, Nob Hill Market (known as Le Beau), an inviting grocery/deli/bakery that has been in this location for 20 years. High-quality produce, as well as fish and other meats, are available. Their take-out sandwiches complement a walk nicely. The mural on the Leavenworth side and another on the Clay side, plus changing art exhibits within the store, attest to the owner's interests and the conviviality of the ambiance.

- ◢ Return to Sacramento, turn left, and walk on the odd-numbered side. The foliage of evenly spaced ficus street trees adds a softness that makes this section of Sacramento inviting.

◢ Turn right into Golden Court. The name *Golden* is on the upper side of the first house. Shrubs of yellow, white, and orange datura are planted on both sides of the walkway. The owner built the gray asbestos-sided house on our right in 1950 (the address is officially No. 1154 Leavenworth) on the only empty lot on the street. He planted the tiglio (known in the U.S. as the linden) tree in 1947 from a seedling his mother brought in her purse from Italy. Golden Court is especially photogenic.

◢ Leroy Place, our next right turn off Sacramento, has two symmetrical rows of ficus trees that frame the walk/cul-de-sac. No. 16 Leroy has attractive bowed windows. Go across Sacramento into the continuation of Leroy. Tall bottlebrush trees on one side and ficus trees on the other enhance the short alley. A basilica-shaped structure at the end of the street is the back of No. 1239 Jones, the Tank High Pressure System of the Fire Department.

◢ We walk out of the cul-de-sac and make a left turn on Sacramento. No. 1315–1325 is a six-flat Edwardian. Continue to Jones.

◢ Grace Episcopal Cathedral School for Boys is on the lower level of the corner of the square block that includes the diocesan house and

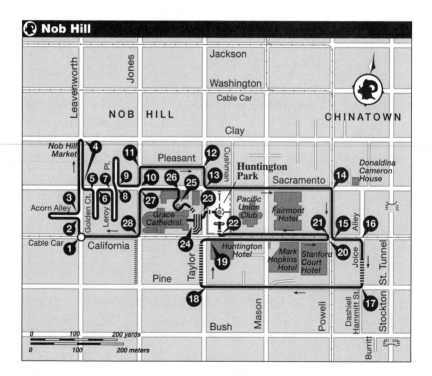

the cathedral itself. You can see the brightly colored playground equipment. The school was built in 1966 for children from kindergarten through eighth grade. Turn left on Jones.

◢ The 1200 and 1300 blocks feature luxury apartments and restaurants: No. 1221 Jones, No. 1250, and the Comstock Apartments at

---

WALK 3 ROUTE: Nob Hill

Public Transportation: California St. Cable Car; MUNI Bus #27 Bryant and #1 California. For MUNI bus information, call 311 (outside San Francisco call (415) 701-2311).

1. Begin at California and Leavenworth. Walk north on Leavenworth to Acorn Alley.
2. Left on Acorn. Return to Leavenworth.
3. Left on Leavenworth to Clay.
4. Return to Sacramento. Left on Sacramento to Golden Court.
5. Right on Golden. Return to Sacramento.
6. Right on Sacramento to Leroy Place.
7. Right on Leroy. Return to Sacramento.
8. Left on Leroy. Return to Sacramento.
9. Left on Sacramento to Jones.
10. Left on Jones to Pleasant.
11. Right on Pleasant to Taylor.
12. Right on Taylor to Sacramento.
13. Left on Sacramento to Powell.
14. Right on Powell to California.
15. Left on California to Joice Alley.
16. Right on Joice. Descend stairway to Pine.
17. Right on Pine to Taylor.
18. Right on Taylor Stwy. to California.
19. Right on California to Powell.
20. Left on Powell.
21. Left on California past Cushman.
22. Ascend stairway into Huntington Park.
23. Descend stairway from the park at Taylor.
24. Cross Taylor. Ascend stairway to Grace Cathedral to explore the interior, labyrinth, and courtyard.
25. Follow walkway across from fountain in the courtyard to Sacramento.
26. Left on Sacramento to Jones.
27. Left on Jones to California.
28. Right on California to your beginning.

No. 1333. Next to No. 1234, turn right into Pleasant. Metrocedros trees line the sidewalk. No. 75 Pleasant has extravagantly large north-facing windows. Across the street is the back of a concrete parking garage. A brass plate on the door of No. 40–44 admonishes: NO SMOKING.

◢ Make a right turn on Taylor. Across the street at No. 1110 is the smallest structure on the block, a one-story, modified, three-window bay, originally built by James Flood, of the Comstock silver mines, for his coachman.

◢ Turn left on Sacramento. No. 1182 has a mailbox at about sidewalk level and a plaque next to it commemorating its Nob Hill architectural award for excellence in 1960. In the sidewalk to the right of No. 1182 Sacramento is a survey monument with the precise latitude and longitude of this spot inscribed under its cover.

◢ Continue east on Sacramento to Powell. You can see cars crossing the Bay Bridge through the narrow opening between skyscrapers. No. 1000 Mason is the elegant Brocklebank Apartments, built in 1924. Ornate mythological beasts are positioned atop the entrance. (Hitchcock's *Vertigo* was filmed here.)

◢ Turn right at Powell to California. The left side of the street is lined with apartments. You can see the octagonal green-and-white, electronically-operated traffic control tower for the cable car system at California and Powell.

◢ Turn left on California to Joice. Ahead at No. 845 is a pleasingly symmetrical Art Deco apartment house with a marble entrance and elaborate light fixtures. Turn right on Joice to the stairway and descend. Two magnolia trees are planted at the first landing. A small shrine to St. Francis is on the lower landing near the graceful curve of the stairs at Pine. The flats, Nos. 738, 740, and 742 Pine are built in the Pueblo style. Across the street is what was once known as Monroe Alley, but is now Dashiell Hammett St. Hammett fans may want to detour to Bush and go into Burritt Alley (between Stockton and Powell) to read the bronze plaque about his novel *The Maltese Falcon*.

◢ Turn right on Pine. At the corner, above the high parapet on the rear of the Stanford Court Hotel, is a cast-stone penguin by Beniamino Bufano, the impecunious artist and bohemian who captured the imagination of San Franciscans and, more importantly, the financial support of patrons in the mid-20th century. At the time of his death in 1970, many of his works were stored in

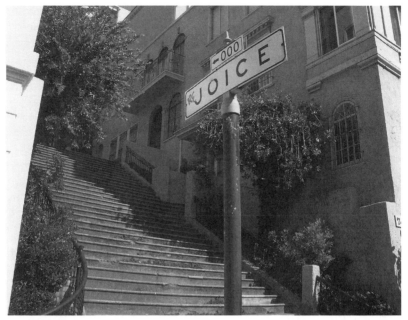

Joice Stairway   *Tony Holiday*

warehouses. Others are scattered in several places: in the courtyard of the Academy of Sciences, at the Phelan St. entrance to the
science building of San Francisco City College, in the meadow at
Fort Mason (Walk 6), on the grounds of the low-cost housing at 370
Valencia, and in the Ordway Building lobby in Oakland.

◢ On Pine, you are now walking along the route of the original
granite retaining wall of the Leland Stanford mansion, which was
destroyed by the earthquake. The blocked entrance in the wall may
have been for tradesmen. The tower with the finial marks the division between the properties of two of the Big Four railroad barons,
Stanford and Mark Hopkins. The wall surrounds these properties
from Pine to California and Powell to Mason.

◢ Turn right on Taylor and ascend the sidewalk stairway to
California. As your bird's-eye view from the top—California
between Taylor and Powell—comes into focus, you see lines of formidable structures: the Fairmont, Mark Hopkins, and Huntington
hotels and the Pacific Union Club. The Stanford Court Hotel
anchors the Powell side; Grace Cathedral and the Cathedral
Apartments are on the Jones side. The secondary line along
Sacramento consists of luxury apartments.

- Turn right on California to the Big Four Restaurant, at No. 1075, in the Huntington Hotel, considered by many one of the City's most elegant hotels. You are welcome to come in between 4 and 5:30 PM to view the panoramic photograph of 1878 San Francisco by Eadweard Muybridge. It is located at the end of the restaurant, to your right.

- Continuing on California, we come to one of my favorites on Nob Hill, No. 1021. Ornate wrought iron double doors provide the entrance to this single-family dwelling; French doors are on the second story. Another favorite is No. 1001, The Morsehead apartment building (1915). Behind the terra-cotta columns and facade are eight apartments, each between 2,000 and 3,000 square feet. The building feels cozier than many on the block.

- Cross Mason to No. 999 California, the Mark Hopkins Hotel, originally the site of the Mark Hopkins home. The hotel opened in 1925. Across Mason, opposite the car entry of the Mark Hopkins Hotel, is a graduated series of town houses, Nos. 831–849 Mason. Designed by Willis Polk around 1918, they provide an imaginative counterfoil to the sumptuous structures on the hill.

When Louis Montesquieu (born in 1689) arrived in a new town, he liked to climb up a high tower to get a good overall look at the place, and then come down and examine the different parts at leisure.

- Turn right and walk down California. Plaques on the side of the Mark Hopkins wall recount some of the site's history. Continue to No. 905, the Stanford Court Hotel, built in 1911. The glass dome is in Aurea restaurant, next to the registration area.

- Continue on California to Powell. Cross Powell and turn left on California. Walk up to Mason to the white granite Fairmont Hotel, at No. 950, which was readied for its grand opening in 1906. On April 18 at 5:15 AM, the fire caused by the earthquake destroyed the interior. Luckily, the fire insurance didn't expire until midnight! The steel frame survived, and a year later the hotel opened for business. A contemporary feature of the Fairmont is the exterior elevator, providing an unusual kinetic experience as you gradually ascend while watching the cityscape.

- As you walk along California, you will see to the right No. 1000, the landmark Pacific Union Club, a private social club with membership by invitation only. James Flood built this brownstone building as his residence in 1886. It is the only one of the mansions on Nob Hill to have survived the fire of 1906 because it was the only one not built of wood. Willis Polk reconstructed and remodeled the home in 1912. The legend that has trickled down through the generations (which we all like to believe, not much caring if it's fact or fiction) says that Flood hired a full-time maintenance man to keep the bronze fence around the property polished.

◢ Continue on California past Cushman to ascend the stairway into Huntington Park. Arabella, the widow of Collis P. Huntington, one of the Big Four railroad barons, donated Huntington Park across the street to the City in 1915. The Huntington home on the property was demolished by the 1906 quake. The park is well designed for both adults and children. The northern section has swings, slides, and a large sandbox. The middle and southern sections feature the Fountain of the Turtles, a delight to contemplate while sitting on the comfortable bench. The Nob Hill Association, in conjunction with Friends of Recreation and Parks, financed a recent renovation of the park and has undertaken the responsibility for maintaining it. Descend the stairway from the park at Taylor and cross the street.

◢ You are now on the block where Charles Crocker, one of the Big Four railroad kings, had built his home. Crocker wanted to own the entire square block. Angered by the audacity of his neighbor who refused to sell his lot at a reasonable price, Crocker built a 40-foot-tall "spite fence" that cut off the sun and view from three sides of Nicholas Yung's home at No. 1203 Sacramento. Yung, a German mortician, was undaunted. He retaliated by putting a curse on Crocker's life, when he built a 10-foot long coffin with a skull and crossbones and positioned it on his roof to face Crocker's house. The 1906 fire demolished both structures. Both men eventually died. Only then were the Crocker heirs able to buy Yung's property from his estate. They subsequently donated the land to the diocese on which the Grace Cathedral complex is located.

◢ Ascend the Grand Stairway to the cathedral that leads you to the magnificent, cast-bronze doors made from the molds of the Renaissance sculptor Lorenzo Ghiberti. High above the doors, you face the rose-window facade of Grace Cathedral.

◢ Traditionally, cathedrals are built over a period of many years. Grace Cathedral is true to this tradition. The cornerstone of Grace Cathedral was laid in 1910; the exterior was completed in 1964;

in 1993, an $11 million construction project completed the design as envisioned by the original architect, Lewis Hobart, who was inspired by Notre Dame. Samuel Yellin executed the subdued, elegant, wrought ironwork on the gates to the Chapel of Grace, on the south side nearest the California St. entrance. Murals by Antonio Sotomayor, chronicling cathedral and parish history, are inside the chapel. (For a better appreciation of the items in the interior, I suggest using one of the self-guided tour pamphlets obtained at the entrance.)

◢ Concerts—sacred, secular, organ, choral, or jazz—are regularly presented. Acoustics are excellent, with a 7- to 12-second delay, depending on the pitch of the instrument. Duke Ellington was commissioned by the diocese to compose a sacred piece, which was performed at a concert in 1965. During the Christmas season of 1990, Bobby McFerrin, the San Francisco singer and conductor, organized a 24-hour sing-a-thon "healing," with various musical groups participating.

◢ To the right of the Grand Stairway is a labyrinth, based on the one at Chartres Cathedral, a tool for meditative walking. Ascend the Bishop Pike Stairway to a wide courtyard, fountain, and cloister. All of these are named for the donors. The Gothic trefoil design repeated on the stained glass windows and the fountain subtlely unites these parts of the grand cathedral complex. Across from the fountain, walk through the cloister to Sacramento.

◢ Turn left on Sacramento to Jones and left on Jones. From here, looking south, you can see the San Bruno Mountain range. At California, near Jones, are a cluster of large apartment and condo buildings—the 1200 Corporation at No. 1200 California, the Cathedral Apartments at No. 1201 California, and the Gramercy Towers condominiums at 1177 California (next to the Masonic Auditorium).

◢ When I think of Nob Hill, I can't help thinking of the wives of the Big Four—Jane Stanford, Arabella Huntington, Elizabeth Hopkins, and Mary Ann Crocker. While their husbands were making decisions in their offices on how to amass millions, these ladies were making decisions in their corporate headquarters (the interiors of their mansions) on how to outdo each other by the millions. *Should I use mahogany for the cabinets or should I wait for the ship from Africa to bring in teak and rosewood? Should I buy that Michelangelo or should I have someone copy it?* Conspicuous consumption merrily reigned. I've never read of any of the wives doing hands-on philanthropic work. How did Mary Ann feel about the spite fence or the skull and crossbones? How did Elizabeth feel about her husband's frugality, his vegetarianism, and his dislike of the ornate furniture she bought? It's difficult to imagine how the wives would have fared if they came west on the Oregon and California trails in covered wagons. Now back to the route.

◢ Turn right on California to Leavenworth to your beginning.

Speaking of

Russian Hill South

Intangibles

Every San Francisco neighborhood has its unique ambiance—a distillation of the folklore and stories of its early days surviving through continual modifications. Russian Hill acquired its name from an early cemetery located on the east side of Vallejo and Jones where Russian sailors were buried before the Gold Rush (a stairway is located on the site). Greek Orthodox crosses and bones have been unearthed there. The sailors had probably come down from Fort Ross, the Russian settlement, with the pelts of seals and otters.

In the late 1800s—and even more so after the 1906 earthquake demolished other structures—small cottages expressing the special ambiance of the neighborhood adorned Russian Hill. The active Russian Hill Neighbors Association is working diligently to preserve this sense of neighborhood in the face of great economic and demographic changes. They have fought the demolition of cottages and their replacement with three- and four-story condominiums. Only about 38 cottages remain out of 100 originally built.

Russian Hill is a craggy, physically compact area. Jasper O'Farrell, the City surveyor, in 1847 extended the street grid to Leavenworth. Somehow, working theoretically and on paper, he didn't make allowance for the hills. As a result of the rectangular street configuration, the summit of Russian Hill became isolated. At Jones a ladder was placed against the bluff to access the 1000 block of Vallejo. Broadway, Vallejo, and Green were impassable for horse teams. These features attracted people who desired a measure of independence with proximity to the City center. The hilltop housing sites made possible the magnificent views, which are still a reason to live on Russian Hill. The topography also encouraged a sense of community among residents. For many years, a large coterie of writers including Bret Harte, George Sterling, and Ina Coolbrith resided on the hill.

◢ Begin at the northeast corner of Polk and Greenwich, where Russian Hill begins its sharp rise toward Larkin. Walk up a partially grooved sidewalk. No. 1342–1344 is a relatively new condominium undergoing another round of exterior painting. The garage has been embellished with a band of decorative ceramic tile placed above its doors.

◢ Turn right on Larkin to Filbert, and then left. The 1200 block of Filbert, from Larkin to Hyde, is composed mostly of Edwardian flats with bay windows on the two upper stories. The block has few trees, but next to No. 1252 is a terraced rock garden. The angled stairway at No. 1234 with its landings appears like a hopscotch diagram. The brown-shingled building at the corner, No. 1205, is designed in the Craftsman style.

◢ Continue past the hum of cables in the slot of Hyde, to walk down the Filbert Stairway. At the bottom of the hill turn right on Leavenworth. In a half block, next to 2033 Leavenworth, you ascend Havens Stairway, a little-known stairway that can only be accessed from Leavenworth (it formerly continued through to Hyde).

◢ The gardens alongside the stairway are cultivated by the property owners living on Havens. The fern garden is one of the most attractive additions to the green space. Return to Leavenworth.

◢ At Leavenworth turn right to Union, then left. Continue to Jones and turn right. Walk into Macondray Lane through a trellised entry into an unexpected garden path, the magical part of Macondray. You see goldfish ponds, garden ornaments, and both annual and perennial plantings. The bordering condos are small but attractive. The area feels as though it ought to be private gardens, but Macondray Lane is a public right-of-way. It is the setting for Armistead Maupin's *Tales of the City*, a television miniseries based on his book of the same name. The variety of trees and shrubs in every shade of green add to the appeal of Macondray Lane, named for a 19th-century merchant and viticulturist.

- Turn back at the cobblestone section. *I do not feel the footing is safe to continue.* Instead, return to Jones.

- Turn right on Jones. Walk to Union, turn right. You will pass a private cul-de-sac alleyway—Marion Place. The plaque gives some of its little known history. Turn right on Taylor and walk to Green. Ascend the stairway on the right to the cul-de-sac, passing an elaborate Art Moderne apartment house on the left, and continue on Green to see an inviting wood-frame house from the 1890s, next to No. 980.

- Towering above everything in sight is No. 999 Green, the Eichler Summit Apartments, built before the height-limitation law was passed in 1970. In the center of the tower, three, long, open, oval shapes like huge exclamation points appear to punctuate the end of a special block, the 1000 block of Green that escaped fire and earthquake damage in 1906.

- Walk to Jones and turn left to enter the arched, double-stairway entrance to a very special section of Vallejo. It is part of Russian Hill's Vallejo St. Crest District, which is on the National Register of Historic Places. You might call this the Livermore section of Vallejo. From 1897 until 2003, some member of the family lived continu-

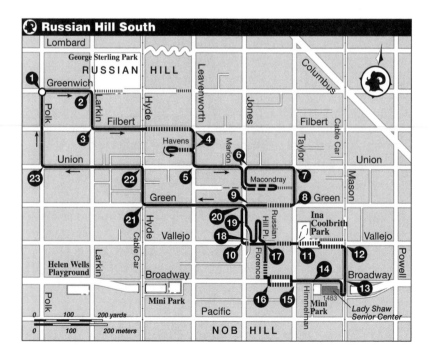

ously in this enclave, staunchly supporting efforts to preserve and maintain the unique character and beauty of the area. You might also call it the Livermore/Polk section. The architect Willis Polk was hired by Horatio Livermore (and later by his son Norman) to build many of the houses and design both the entrance on Jones and the stairway to Taylor.

WALK 4 ROUTE: Russian Hill South

Public Transportation: MUNI Bus #19 Polk; #47 and #49 Van Ness. For MUNI bus information, call 311 (outside San Francisco call (415) 701-2311).

1. Begin at Polk and Greenwich.
2. Right on Larkin to Filbert.
3. Left on Filbert. Descend sidewalk stairway to Leavenworth.
4. Right on Leavenworth. Ascend Havens Stwy. and return to Leavenworth. Turn right.
5. Left on Union to Jones.
6. Right to Macondray Lane. Left to explore and return. Right to Union. Right to Taylor.
7. Right to Green.
8. Ascend Green Stwy. to Jones.
9. Left on Jones to Vallejo.
10. Left onto Vallejo Stwy. into cul-de-sac, walk to end.
11. Descend Vallejo Stwy. next to No. 1019, past Taylor to Mason.
12. Right on Mason. Cross Broadway to see Lady Shaw Senior Center at No. 1483 Mason.
13. Cross back to Broadway; left (west) on Broadway.
14. Continue on Broadway past Himmelman Place Mini Park.
15. Continue west on sidewalk stairway past Taylor to Florence.
16. Ascend Florence Stwy.
17. Walk across Vallejo into Russian Hill Place.
18. Right to walk down ramp to Jones.
19. Right on Jones to Green.
20. Left on Green to Hyde.
21. Right on Hyde to Union.
22. Left on Union to Polk.
23. Right on Polk to Greenwich to your beginning.

Linking

If you wish to link Russian Hill South with Russian Hill North (Walk 5), begin at Polk and Lombard and follow the directions in Walk 5.

- Continue to the end of the cul-de-sac, walking on the odd-numbered south side. No. 1023 is the Horatio Livermore house, built by Julia Morgan in 1917. A developer demolished three red-wood-shingled houses at No. 1030, designed by Joseph Worcester circa 1889. They have since been replaced by the Hermitage condominium apartments, which duplicate the Craftsman style so appropriate for the nooks and crannies of Russian Hill. The architects Joseph Worcester, Julia Morgan, Bernard Maybeck, Willis Polk, and Ernest Coxhead built homes in this style during the first quarter of the 20th century as an antidote to the excesses and formalism of Victorian architecture. They emphasized natural elements: redwood shingles and protruding eaves instead of bracketed cornices and gabled roofs. Trees and shrubs were an important part of the design, and homes were designed to blend harmoniously with the topography.

- Polk (1867–1924) designed No. 1019 for the artist Doris Williams (notice the high, half-moon window in her north-facing studio). As part of his fee, he was given the adjoining lot. Here he built No. 1013 for himself in 1892. The house drops down through six levels and is now divided into three apartments.

- In 1915 Laura Ingalls Wilder, who wrote the Little House series (the best known volume of which is *Little House on the Prairie*), came to San Francisco to see the Panama-Pacific International Exposition. She stayed with her daughter, Rose, a feature writer for the *San Francisco Bulletin*, who lived at No. 1019. Laura wrote letters home to her husband in Missouri about the fair, the City, the people, and life on Russian Hill. These letters have been collected in a small paperback titled *West from Home*.

Horatio Gates Livermore walked from St. Joseph, Missouri, to San Francisco in 1850.

- The Open Space at the top of the hill was the 50-vara lot (a California *vara* roughly equals 33 inches) that Horatio Livermore bought in 1889. In 1914, after the residents had subscribed $25,000 for the balustrades and ramps that Polk designed on the Jones side, the top of the summit became the carriage turnaround.

- The story of the Polk-designed Vallejo Stairway, which you descend, is one of concerted effort by neighbors over a period of many years to beautify and maintain the surrounding gardens.

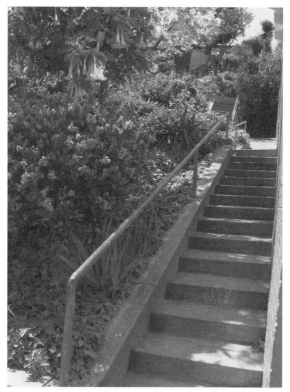

Vallejo Stairway   *Adah Bakalinsky*

To continue within the historic context of the neighborhood, they replaced 14 replicas of early lamps (now with halogen bulbs) and installed benches for resting and viewing. This project was the inspiration for the Los Angeles Los Feliz neighborhood major stairway and ceramic mural wall renovation.

⏍ Enter the Ina Coolbrith Park (dedicated in 1911), across the street from No. 1715 Taylor, to descend to Mason. Ina Coolbrith (1841–1928), whose uncle Joseph Smith founded the Mormon Church, came to San Francisco from Illinois at the age of 10 in the first covered-wagon train that crossed the Sierra via Beckwourth Pass. She taught school and later became a librarian at the Bohemian Club and the Oakland Public Library. Although she was honored as poet laureate of California in 1915, her main contribution to the San Francisco literary world was as a catalyst to aspiring writers. Joaquin Miller, George Sterling, Bret Harte, Gelett Burgess, and others met regularly at her home (1067 Broadway) for readings.

- Many elderly Chinese come to the park daily to practice Tai Chi. Their mental concentration and slow body movements echo the harmony conveyed by the surrounding canopy of Monterey pines.

- At Mason you're on the edge of Chinatown and Russian Hill. Turn right for one block, then right again on Broadway. Notice how the land dips and rises, extending to the highest point south, Nob Hill (Walk 3).

- You are now above the Broadway Tunnel, which extends under Russian Hill from Mason to Larkin. Although the tunnel was proposed in 1874 to facilitate the flow of traffic, it opened for vehicular traffic in 1952—78 years later!

- Walk across Broadway to No. 1483 Mason to see the 69-unit Lady Shaw Senior Center, completed in late 1990. The center was financed by her husband, Sir Run Run Shaw, and his brother, Run Me Shaw, through their Shaw Foundation, which supports education, welfare, medicine, and the arts, with a particular emphasis on aiding the elderly, and is one of the largest foundations in the world. Building above the tunnel was controversial, but the critical need for housing in Chinatown, the fine design by architect Gordon Chong & Associates, and the infusion of private, city, and federal funding were decisive factors in favor of construction.

- Return to Broadway and turn left. At No. 906, you will see the twin-towered former Spanish National Church, Nuestra Señora de Guadalupe. The 1912 structure is built on the site of the original 1875 wood church.

- At the northwest corner of Broadway and Taylor, there is a high retaining wall with decorative edging along the top. Grading of the slopes in the 1860s and 1870s created vertical bluffs. When the streets were lowered, retaining walls and stairways became necessary to protect the houses perched on the top. Walk up the sidewalk stairway on the south side of Broadway for a better view of No. 1020, located up high and toward the back of the property. This two-story, brown-shingle, Craftsman-style house was designed by Albert Farr in 1909.

- Ascend the Florence Stairway next to No. 1032 Broadway. The concrete wall topped with spindle decoration and the brass plaque (sometimes under cascading vines) states ATKINSON-NICHOLS LANDMARK BUILDING—1858. There's something strange about this stairway: As you approach each landing, the landscape also seems to rise. Nos. 35, 37, and 39 Florence are Pueblo Revival–style with stucco exteriors and deep-set window apertures to deflect the sun. Robert A. Stern has redesigned No. 40, the original Livermore house on Florence.

⊿ When you reach Vallejo (Gelett Burgess lived at No. 1071 for three years), cross the street into Russian Hill Place. Nos. 1, 3, 5, and 7 Russian Hill Place, designed by Willis Polk, were built for Norman Livermore in 1913. It's hard to believe that Russian Hill possesses such a concentration of bewitching little streets in such a small area!

⊿ Return to Vallejo and turn right to walk down the ramp to Jones; turn right to Green, and make a left turn. Walk on the south side, the odd-numbered side. The 1000 block of Green was spared from the earthquake and fire of 1906, so it's architecturally notable. No. 1039–43 is an Italianate of the 1880s and was moved here after 1906. No. 1040 was once the home of the Folger family, whose fortune was made from importing, roasting, and packaging coffee. No. 1055 dates from 1866 and was later remodeled by Julia Morgan. The beautiful carriage house at the rear is now used as living quarters. You can also see the 1857 octagon house, the oldest in the City, at No. 1067. A cupola was added in the 1880s. Octagon houses were in vogue for a while because they were purported to be beneficial to your health and sexual vigor. (If you wish to tour the interior of an octagon house, check the hours of the Colonial Dames Octagon at 2645 Gough or call (415) 441-7512.) Engine Company No. 31 formerly occupied the 1907 Tudor Revival–style firehouse across the street, which is now a National Trust property.

⊿ When you reach Hyde, turn right and then left on Union, the center of the neighborhood shopping area. Across the street, No. 1200 Hyde was Home Drug, where various members of the same family operated the store from 1911 to 1994. The Searchlight Market has been here for 100 years under various owners. The original Swensen's Ice Cream, here since 1948, still makes the sweet treat on the premises. These shopkeepers provide continuity and stability that contribute to the intangible that is Russian Hill.

⊿ Continue west on Union to Polk, and turn right to Greenwich to your beginning.

San Francisco

RUSSIAN HILL NORTH

Architectural

Signatures

From the vantage point of Pacific Heights, Russian Hill appears to be shaped like a square-toed shoe. Coincidentally, many sections of Russian Hill are accessible only to walkers. The redwood-shingled, Craftsman-style homes, designed by Northern California architects Julia Morgan, Willis Polk, and Bernard Maybeck in the early 1900s, blend well into this terrain. Irregularly shaped, deep lots abound; some houses—the kind I call "tuck-ins"—are almost invisible from the street. These tuck-ins are as much a part of the City's architectural signature as the loftier towers you see on this walk.

◢ We begin at the corner of Polk and No. 1299 Lombard, built in 1928. The eye-catching ceramic-tiled step risers, decorative metal on the doors, and bas-relief on the pillars provide a dramatic beginning to our exploration of the neighborhood. The 1200 block of Lombard beautifully illustrates the congeniality between the interspersed Italianates and Craftsman-style homes, and between the homes and their hillside location. In this block are several "invisibles," homes that are landlocked and better seen from across the street. Cross Lombard to view No. 1275, a large shingled Italianate, and Nos. 1267–1263, redwood-shingled refurbished Victorians of 1877. Nos. 1249–1251, a San Francisco Stick Italianate, is a beautiful flat-front tuck-in with a staircase. Built on a hill, it is doubly imposing with its tall false front. No. 1257 is truly a tuck-in and almost hidden. These were all built in the years 1877–1878.

In 1821 at the age of 60, Adam Link walked from his home in Pennsylvania to Ohio (141 miles in 3 days).

◢ Opposite No. 1251 Lombard descend the Culebra Terrace Stairway. The hard-to-see sign is on the side of No. 1250. This is a stairway with 29 steps, three landings, and a coda of two steps.

◢ Culebra Terrace is a charming alley of flats and single dwellings enhanced by trees, shrubbery, and flowers. What gives the alley cohesiveness is the combination and proximity of house colors that interact with one another from shades of terracotta to yellow. Built in 1911, No. 23 is one of the oldest in the alley. No. 35 has the simplicity of a child's drawing of a house and window. No. 50 has a curved second story of five windows. No. 60 has a terrazzo stairway and decorative small tiles that you see from the glass door. But as you look at the exterior, you may see a sculpted dragonfly high in the middle of the wall. The smaller one is on the lower right-hand side of the wall. The creator of the sculpture is Arthur McLaughlin. You emerge from Culebra onto the Chestnut cul-de-sac. Across the street is No. 1154 Chestnut, a villa built in 1913 by a Canadian silver mine owner. Two curved stairways, with wrought iron railings, partially encircle a flowing fountain that predominates the entrance to the house. This is purported to be the first residence in San Francisco that used steel reinforced concrete for its structure. There are four sycamore street trees planted in front of the house.

◢ This house has historical significance. It was the residence of the Edwin and Irma Grabhorn for 50 years. The Grabhorn Press of San Francisco was and is still considered one of the finest small letter presses in the world. After the death of the Grabhorn brothers, the Grabhorn Institute was organized in 2000. The Institute has been recognized with a California Heritage Council Award in 2002 for "preservation of the last fully functioning type foundry and integrated letterpress printing facility."

- The Institute was also recognized for its work to preserve the type-casting and letterpress printing operation of Arion Press and M & H Type by the National Trust for Historic Preservation as part of "the nation's irreplaceable historical and cultural legacy" under its Save America's Treasures program. Tours are given on Thursdays at 3 PM. The fee is $7. Contact them at (415) 668-2542 for reservations.

- As we turn to ascend the stairway, we see on our right a building, No. 1141, designed with a four-story series of angled sections built to maximize sun and views for the residents.

- Walk up the wide Chestnut Stairway shadowed by Canary Island pines and Italian stone pines. Neighbors are working on the land-scaping. Forty-eight steps bring you to a landing where a U-shaped double stairway begins. From the landing you see one of two dominant landmarks of that part of the City—the unmistakable dome of the Palace of Fine Arts (Walk 8). Walk up the left stairway

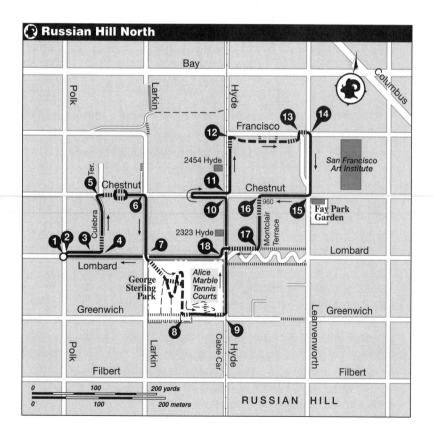

to Larkin. Looking back down the Chestnut corridor, you can see the Presidio on the northwest side of San Francisco.

◢ Turn right on Larkin. An apartment house on the corner has a brass plaque: 2677 LARKIN AT CHESTNUT. (Unfortunately, the architect's name and the date are not cited.)

◢ Continue one block to Lombard. At the corner walk up the stairway into George Sterling Park, named for the poet who lived on Russian Hill during the 1920s. He is remembered for his description of San Francisco as the "cool gray city of love." Two plaques about him are located at the bottom of the stairway. The low-lying trunks of leptospermum trees and the nodules of exposed roots

---

WALK 5 ROUTE: Russian Hill North

Public Transportation: MUNI Bus #19 Polk; #47 and #49 Van Ness. For MUNI bus information, call 311 (outside San Francisco call (415) 701-2311).

1. Begin at Polk and Lombard, right side of street at No. 1299 Lombard.
2. Cross Lombard to walk up left (north) side of the street.
3. Continue to Culebra Terrace sign at No. 1250.
4. Descend Culebra Terrace Stwy.
5. Right up Chestnut Stwy. to Larkin.
6. Right on Larkin. Continue on Larkin to Lombard.
7. Ascend stairway to George Sterling Park. Bear left on path to Greenwich Stwy.
8. Left on stairway to Hyde.
9. Left on Hyde to Lombard. Continue to Chestnut.
10. Detour to 1000 block of Chestnut to view architecture of houses.
11. Return to Hyde and turn left.
12. Right at Francisco. Walk on right upper pedestrian sidewalk toward Leavenworth.
13. Descend stairway. Turn left and descend opposite stairway to Leavenworth.
14. Right on Leavenworth to Chestnut.
15. Right on Chestnut to No. 960.
16. Ascend stairway to Montclair Terrace and continue to Lombard.
17. Right turn on Lombard. Ascend sidewalk stairway to Hyde.
18. Continue on Lombard to Polk to your beginning.

Linking

If you wish to link Russian Hill North with Russian Hill South (Walk 4), begin at Polk and Greenwich and follow the directions in Walk 4.

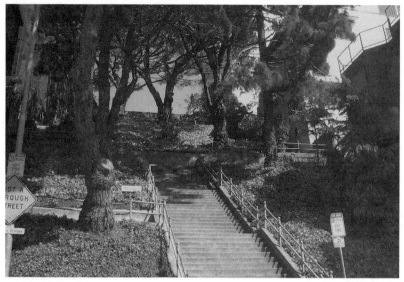

Chestnut Stairway *Tony Holiday*

along the path give you a feeling of entering ancient woods. A bench has been thoughtfully placed to permit a meditative view northwest to the Marin hills.

◢ Bear left up the stairs past the bench (to the sound above of tennis balls against racquets). The next landing is Phoebe's Terrace (named for a neighborhood benefactor). Pass the mosaic tile wall, and then walk right on the sidewalk. Watch for posted signs: BE COYOTE AWARE. The white crown sparrows seem to have the air rights around here. Perfect acoustics for their beautiful song, and perfect sighting for their gliding and dipping flights. Tennis and basketball players gradually come into view on the left. A plaque for Phoebe Terrace is on the concrete post as you approach the Greenwich Stairway.

◢ Turn left to ascend the stairway and explore the stone terraced ramps and landscaping leading to the tennis courts. This park was restored in 2005 by the San Francisco Public Utilities Commission.

◢ The Alice Marble Tennis Courts, also part of the 2.6-acre park, are on Water Department land, with the Lombard reservoir beneath (built in 1860) supplying six to eight surrounding blocks. Born in the small California town of Dutch Flat, Alice Marble (1913–1990) spent some of her adolescent years in San Francisco. She joined the Golden Gate Park Tennis Club, a training ground for many outstanding players and, during 1936–1940, was a four-time winner of the National Women's Singles Tennis championship. A plaque tells of the rededication of the reservoir to her in 2005.

⚐ Descend 26 steps to Hyde, turn left facing Alcatraz (another San Francisco signature), and continue to Lombard. No. 2222 is an eight-story steel-framed, reinforced-concrete cooperative (1920), one of five constructed by T. Paterson Ross in the Russian Hill neighborhood. His buildings are rich in interior detail and utilize the latest technology of their era of construction. Ross designed about 200 buildings during a 32-year period. When he sustained brain injuries from falling bricks in an open freight elevator while inspecting the Union League Club, his professional career ended. He was 49 then but lived to be 84.

⚐ The intersection of Hyde and Lombard is a splendid place to stop and see the Hyde Street Cable Car lurching along with its standing-room-only crowd of passengers. Accorded the conductor's full approval, they alight en masse with their cameras pointed toward Alcatraz, Coit Tower, the Bay Bridge, or Treasure Island. At the clang of the cable car bell, they rush aboard once more to coast down to the next landing on their way to Aquatic Park. No. 2323 Hyde, across the street, is a Willis Polk house designed for Robert Louis Stevenson's widow, Fanny, who lived there from 1899 to 1908. (Lombard and Hyde was purported to be Stevenson's favorite San Francisco corner.) The structure is now an apartment house.

⚐ Continue walking north on Hyde to Chestnut. An inappropriately placed high-rise on the corner still suffers that friendless look. Previously this was the site (No. 998 Chestnut) of the landmark 12-room house built in 1852 by William Clark, who built the first wharf near the foot of Broadway (Walk 1).

⚐ Detour left on Chestnut to experience the ambiance of the 1000 block. Between Nos. 1000 and 1080 is a delightful series of three-story, mansard-roofed homes painted in pastel colors. The south side of the street features the back entrance of the award-winning Lombardia complex, 10 large town houses and 32 condos designed by well-known architects Hood and Miller (on a lot that was vacant for 28 years). By thoughtful use of scale, space, light, and plant materials, they created an inviting Mediterranean setting. No. 1089 Chestnut, completed in 1990, has 17-foot ceilings in the living room and 5,600 square feet of space.

- Return to Hyde, turn left (north), and walk on the right side of the street past the Norwegian Seaman's Church at No. 2454 Hyde. From the left side of Hyde you can see the roof of another reservoir. Straight ahead (north) is the Hyde St. Pier with its famous collection of historic ships. At Francisco turn right and walk on the upper pedestrian sidewalk toward Leavenworth.

- The Francisco cul-de-sac is one of my favorites. The large homes here, designed in a variety of architectural styles, are set on several levels of land to command enviable views from either side of the street.

- The frame two-story at No. 825 is originally dated 1849 but has undergone many renovations. It was constructed of timber salvaged from ships abandoned in the Bay during the Gold Rush. No. 828 Francisco, at the end of the cul-de-sac, has a bay of leaded windows with octagonal inserts, a modified mansard roof, and beautiful copper chimney stacks, which have acquired a greenish cast over the years. A fence espaliered with jasmine follows the slope of the hill.

- From the parapet next to No. 800 Francisco, you can gaze at the variety of geometric shapes and signatures that are part of a San Franciscan's daily eyeful: the abundant, sword-shaped leaves of a

Vallejo Stairway *Tony Holiday*

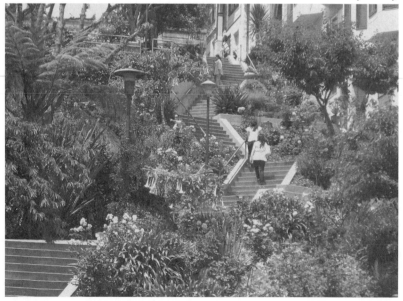

palm tree at the lower corner of the street, the square Romanesque tower of the San Francisco Art Institute, the rectangular towers of the Bay Bridge, the conical towers of Saints Peter and Paul Church in North Beach, the cylindrical Coit Tower, and the pyramidal Transamerica building.

- Descend the short stairway to the street. Cross to the opposite side of Francisco and descend the stairway to Leavenworth. Walk across Leavenworth and turn right to Chestnut. At the corner of Leavenworth, detour a few steps to Fay Park Garden at No. 2366 Leavenworth. San Francisco was the recent recipient of this property owned by the Fay family. It is distinguished by a Thomas Church garden that was designed for the family in 1957 and includes trees, flowers, and gazebos. The garden is now open to the public; however, the mansion is not, at this time.

- Turn right on Chestnut. No. 930 has a flat roof, while No. 944, built in 1864, has columns and a balcony. Across the street from No. 960, ascend 28 steps to Montclair Terrace, a hidden court of homes and gardens. No. 66, designed in 1956 by one of my favorite architects, Henry Hill, has simplicity and flourish. Next to No. 4 you're at Lombard, where drivers enjoy the unusual ride down the most photographed, photogenic, hairpin-turn street in the country: eight turns within an 800-foot-long section with a grade of 18.18%. City engineer Preston Wallace King designed it in 1922, from a 26% grade, cobblestoned Lombard.

- Turn right on Lombard to walk up a straight, comfortable stairway. At the top, continue west on Lombard to Polk to your beginning.

Metamorphosis

Fort Mason

in Action

In Fort Mason (named for the first military gov-
ernor of California, Richard Barnes Mason), an
area of about 89 acres, you can trace a continuously
evolving historical line from 1797 to the present, from
Spanish and American military fortifications to a section of
the Golden Gate National Recreation Area (GGNRA). The
integration of history and land-use objectives is resulting in a
unification of the past and present. For instance, as military artifacts
from the past are unearthed, they are placed for viewing in contextual
areas, necessitating the redesign of spaces and trails. More recent history is also being commemorated: The Phillip Burton Memorial was
relandscaped to accommodate better viewing of the sculpture, green
spaces, and new paths.

On this walk you explore some of the extensive municipal and federal recreational areas of San Francisco along the northern waterfront.
Walking west from Marina Green through Presidio lands or east from
the Marina Green to the Hyde St. Pier, you can appreciate how this
land became a focus for federal military installations, and then slowly
evolved, under the aegis of the Department of the Interior, into land
for a national park. The area you traverse is part of the GGNRA, the
most popular urban park in the United States. More apparent here
than in other neighborhoods is how the continuum of past history
blends into an evolving contemporary scene. Naturally, the atmosphere is highly energized.

The most propitious time to go on the Fort Mason walk is in the morning—a sunny, windless morning. If you arrive by car, park either at Gashouse Cove or the Marina Green parking area. There is a fee to park in the Fort Mason parking lot.

◢ Begin on the Gashouse Cove Marina path and enter Fort Mason by the side of Bldg. A. (Pick up a calendar of events at the Fort Mason Foundation office, or call (415) 441-3400.) For many years this was the point of embarkation for men and supplies. The Army used the buildings alongside the piers through demobilization after World War II and the Korean conflict. They are now used for recreational and cultural activities. Lower Fort Mason, which is managed and administered by the nonprofit Fort Mason Foundation, is the headquarters for more than 50 nonprofit community and cultural organizations. These organizations include theaters, museums, music schools, dance classes, computer groups, the Children's Art Center, and Lawyers for the Arts. The Greens Restaurant in Bldg. A, an outstanding vegetarian restaurant, has been here since 1979. The restaurant seating offers a view of the Bay and Golden Gate Bridge.

◢ Walk toward the water and then to your right. You pass Bldgs. A, B, C, D, and E; Pier 1; Pier 2, Herbst Pavilion, and Cowell Theater; and Pier 3, Festival Pavilion. Along these buildings and piers there are working Exploratorium exhibits. The J. Porter Shaw Maritime Library in Bldg. E is open to the general public Monday through Friday by appointment; call (415) 561-7030. As you walk along the wall, note the stern of *The Galilee*, a Tahitian trading vessel, built in 1891 and in use until 1920. The Oceanic Society has its offices nearby.

◢ Opposite Bldg. E is a stairway. As I walked up the first series of steps, I saw hummingbirds dipping and revolving around one another in their courtship ritual. A Monterey cypress is on the left.

◢ The next level at Fort Mason features former military housing, the International Hostel, and the GGNRA headquarters—a resource for information about the entire national park system as well as community conservation issues. (For more information, call (415) 561-4700.) The Park Service continually monitors problem areas. They plant soil-huggers like sand verbena, ice plant, and dune daisy to restrain the constantly shifting, sandy soil. They build stairways to prevent erosion, preserve the fragile topsoil, and keep people on the trails.

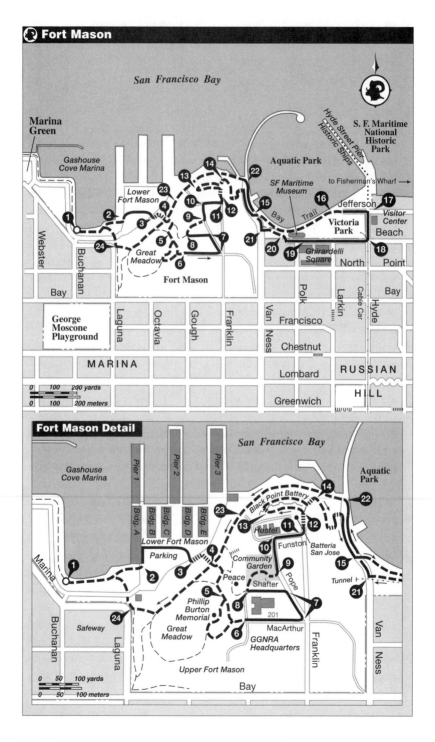

- Turn around to see Marina Blvd., the Golden Gate Bridge, and the Marin Headlands.

- Take the path to the left, walking counterclockwise toward the Great Meadow. You are retracing the long-forgotten footsteps of hundreds of men, women, and children who lived here in tents after losing their homes in the 1906 earthquake. Refugee Camp

---

WALK 6 ROUTE: Fort Mason

Public Transportation: MUNI Bus #28 19th Ave. For MUNI bus information, call 311 (outside San Francisco call (415) 701-2311).

Parking: Available at Gashouse Cove or Marina Green, as well as inside the gate at Fort Mason for a fee.

1. Begin at Gashouse Cove.
2. Walk on sidewalk along waterfront to the side of Bldg. A in lower Fort Mason.
3. Ascend the stairway opposite Bldg. E.
4. Walk on any of the paths around or through the Great Meadow.
5. Pass Bufano sculpture *Madonna.* Pass Phillip Burton Memorial.
6. Left on MacArthur to Park Headquarters (Bldg. No. 201).
7. Left on Pope. Left at Bldg. 204.
8. Walk around Community Gardens and out on Pope.
9. Left on Pope.
10. Right on Funston.
11. Left on Franklin.
12. Walk to the end of Franklin and descend stairway.
13. Left and walk around Black Point Battery. Ascend wood stairway to upper level.
14. Right on footpath at top of wall. Descend stairways and walkways to Van Ness. Turn right.
15. Cross Van Ness. Turn right and then left on promenade.
16. Continue on promenade to Jefferson and Hyde.
17. Right on Hyde to Beach.
18. Right on Beach to Polk.
19. Continue across Polk and past the Maritime Museum. Veer left past low white wall and benches.
20. Descend stairway. Turn left and walk railroad-track path to Van Ness.
21. Right on Van Ness to the pier.
22. At pier, turn left to ascend paved path.
23. Follow path through Great Meadow to Laguna.
24. At bottom of hill, across from Safeway, you are at your beginning.

No. 5 extended west beyond the meadow to the site of the present Safeway store. Fort Mason was an important site during and after the 1906 earthquake. The Navy fireboat anchored here was used to pump water from the Bay to the fire engines along Van Ness. Fort Mason was the headquarters for General Frederick Funston, who had to put San Francisco under martial law to prevent looting. Subsequently, under General Adolphus Washington Greely, it became the relief-supply distribution center. When Mayor Eugene Schmitz moved his office here, Fort Mason became the center for coordinating civil and military authority.

◢ Following the paved footpath to the right, you reach the Beniamino Bufano sculpture of cast stone and mosaic dedicated to and named *Madonna*. A favorite San Francisco personality, Bufano (1898–1970) was supported by various benefactors, such as the owner of the Powell restaurant (now defunct) for which he designed and executed a mosaic mural in return for a lifetime of meals.

◢ Walk along the path to the Phillip Burton Memorial, designed by landscape architect Tito Patri; the project sculptor was Wendy Ross. The 10-foot sculpture of Burton represents him in his everyday look—rumpled trousers, emphatic gesture, and a scribbled note in his jacket pocket. In 1983, Congress dedicated the GGNRA to Congressman Burton, who was responsible for the federal legislation that made the park a reality. The sculpture was unveiled in the spring of 1991. (If you look to the right, you can see the Palace of Fine Arts dome and Golden Gate Bridge.)

◢ Continue east on the path to Park Headquarters, Bldg. No. 201, on MacArthur Street. It was built in 1901 as a military hospital. After the 1906 earthquake, it was used as an emergency center and a lying-in hospital. According to legend, eight babies were born at Fort Mason the night after the quake.

◢ In the years following 1906, Bldg. No. 201 was used as administrative headquarters for Fort Mason. During World War II Ronald Reagan (president of the United States, 1981–1989) served here as second lieutenant in charge of tracking down missing shipments. Fort Mason was declared a National Historic Landmark in 1985.

◢ Make a sharp left turn on Pope to pass around headquarters. To your right, near the corner of Franklin, are the Mission Revival–style Chapel (1942) and the starting place of the Conversation-Pace Game field, sponsored by the San Francisco Senior Center. Various exercises here are paced slowly enough to allow for conversation.

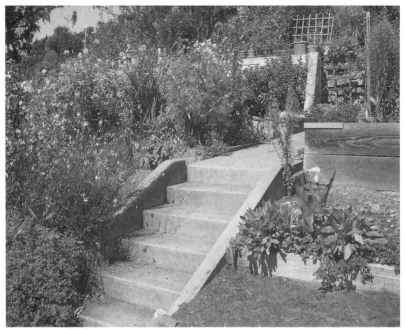

Fort Mason Community Garden   *Tony Holiday*

⬛ Continue on Pope past Shafter. At Bldg. 204 turn left on the sidewalk into the gated Community Garden to explore greenhouses, lattice works, and terraces, and view the enormous variety of plants, vegetables, and flowers in cultivation. Several gardeners specialize in rare varieties of flowers. The Fort Mason garden is very popular and, even though space is available to anyone who applies, the average wait time is five years. Return to Pope, and go left.

⬛ The San Francisco International Hostel at the end of Pope, Bldg. 240, formerly a Civil War barracks built in 1863, is a friendly, clean, and inviting place. You may see some of the guests lolling about on the grass, while others may be reading. The hostel can accommodate 151, including nine private rooms; there is 24-hour access and no curfew.

⬛ From the hostel turn right on Funston, passing the sign for Bldg. 240. Continue to Franklin and walk across to the area interpretive sign. This part of Fort Mason contains military residences dating from the 1850s. The officers' housing on the east side of Pope originated as squatters' homes, put up in the same period by prominent

San Franciscans who understood the value of the real estate. Shortly afterward the Army took possession of the homes and began building up fortifications in anticipation of a Confederate attack.

◢ Strong pro- and anti-slavery feelings in California culminated in the famous Terry-Broderick duel in 1859. Senator David Broderick, shot by the hot-tempered, pro-slavery Judge David Terry near Lake Merced, died here at Fort Mason in the home of a friend. The Haskell House interpretive sign is to the right.

◢ Continue left on Franklin along the concrete walkway. You pass the Palmer House erected in 1855. Then you reach an open green space on the left, where John Fremont's home was from 1859 to 1861. The upper area was also the site of the Batteria San Jose, a Spanish seacoast defense battery located here in 1797. It was built to protect the Yerba Buena anchorage, later known as Black Point Cove (1820s) and now known as Aquatic Park. Black Point Cove was once part of the San Jose Point Military Reservation, which became Fort Mason in 1882.

◢ This particular area of land was important to the Spanish, Mexicans, and Americans because of its strategic location for defense. Theoretically, the Bay was well defended against hostile fleets. At one time or another there were Spanish or American coastal batteries on the Marin Headlands, Alcatraz, Angel Island, Fort Point, and here at Fort Mason. The best preserved of these antiquated defenses is Fort Point, the Civil War fort under the arch of the Golden Gate Bridge.

◢ Walk to the end of Franklin and descend the stairway to the picnic area and Black Point Battery. You are standing on what is known as Black Point Lookout, so-called because of the dark vegetation provided by the laurel trees. The picnic area was constructed on this battery platform, which dates to the Civil War. There are four tables and benches where you can sit to enjoy food and the sublime view, which, when I visited, featured a procession of boats with multicolored sails of pink, green, and blue, backlit against the clearly delineated hills of Marin and the East Bay. Reservations must be made for use of the tables by calling (415) 561-4300.

◢ Walk across the area of the battery emplacements in the wall on your left. At the western end there is a 10-ton cannon. The sign reads 1863 BATTERY. Another emplacement sign reads 1898 BATTERY, both part of Black Point Battery. This site was excavated from 1981 to 1983. The land is stabilized with no further excavations planned. To your left is a native plant habitat in the process of being planted. Ascend the railroad-tie steps to the wall of the battery. Turn right and walk back to the picnic area.

◢ Turn left to descend the stairway. As you turn right to walk the long, paved walkway, these are some of the sights that come into view: East Bay; both structures of the Oakland Bay Bridge connected by Yerba Buena Island; Treasure Island identified as the long strip of land left of Yerba Buena; Fisherman's Wharf; the long pedestrian pier at the end of Van Ness; the Cannery; Hyde Street Pier with historic ships. Continue on the walkway, where concrete and stone benches have conveniently been placed. When you pass a gate that leads to a private residence, bear left down the stairways and walkway to Van Ness.

◢ Cross the extension of Van Ness to be on the waterside along Aquatic Park. Public restrooms are located in the white structure with incised wavy lines near the roofline to simulate ocean waves, an example of the Streamline Moderne style of the 1930s. (The twin of this one is located at the end of Jefferson.) Take the walkway just before the public restrooms. Walk on the promenade along the water and ascend the amphitheater steps to watch birds and swimmers. The inviting sandy beach we enjoy today was originally a dismal beach of gravel and seaweed. It was renovated with tons of sand taken from Union Square when the underground garage was built in the 1930s.

Samuel Taylor Coleridge walked 10 miles daily and worked out the setting of The Rime of the Ancient Mariner *on a walking tour with William Wordsworth.*

◢ The ship-shaped building to the right, originally Aquatic Park Bathhouse, a WPA project of 1939, is now the Maritime Museum founded by Karl Kortum in 1950. Restored murals located on the street level floor are available for viewing. The Aquatic Park Senior Center, active since 1947, uses part of the building. The first and second floors of the museum are open from 10 AM to 4 PM daily. The third floor, at this time, is closed.

◢ Walk east on Jefferson, passing the Dolphin Swimming and Boating Club established in 1877. Members still swim in the Bay. Next to it is the South End Rowing Club.

- Historic ships are docked at the Hyde St. Pier, and one can take an imaginary trip: on the *Eureka*, a passenger ferry; the *Thayer*, a sailing schooner that carried lumber, salmon, and codfish; and the *Balclutha*, a square-rigger. A nominal fee to board the ships helps defray the expense of preserving them. The bookstore has an excellent collection pertaining to the sea and related subjects.

- At the corner of Hyde and Jefferson, cross the street to the San Francisco Maritime National Historical Park Visitor Center. Here are exhibits of local maritime history. It opens daily at 9:30 AM and is staffed by park rangers. You may enjoy a visit next door to the cannery for shopping and browsing.

- Walk up Hyde along the side of Victoria Park (designed by Thomas Church in 1960), which is festive with a gazebo and flowers, and the Cable Car turntable. Jovial crowds of tourists and residents wait to board.

- Turn right on Beach. Musicians and performers are interspersed among the outdoor stall displays of jewelry, T-shirts, leather belts, pen and ink drawings of San Francisco scenes, and stained-glass mobiles and window insets.

- Continue to Larkin. Ghirardelli Square, at the corner, is a pioneer example of adaptive use. In this case, the former chocolate factory, which was built in 1893, was converted in 1967 into a well-designed complex of residences, fine-quality specialty shops, and restaurants.

- Continue on Beach and cross Polk. Walk past the Maritime Museum and the low wall and benches. Descend the stairway to the promenade. Turn left on the railroad-track path back to Van Ness. Across the street is the tunnel, bored into the rocks under Fort Mason, through which the Belt Line Railroad tracks ran. The Belt Line, opened in 1896, covered the City front from Islais Creek to the Presidio. The original purpose was to move boxcars and flatcars directly alongside cargo vessels. In the late 1920s, men and military supplies were transported to the Presidio; in the late 1950s the military filled the tracks.

- Turn right on Van Ness and walk along the curved concrete wall of Aquatic Park to the pier. Pumping Station No. 2, built to supply water in case of earthquake and fire, is on the left side of the street. Opposite, you can see the small, fenced wood section of what was formerly the Alcatraz Pier. Here, convicts boarded a boat for the island prison.

- Turn left and walk up the paved path to the Great Meadow, where additional Exploratorium exhibits have been placed. Along the way you will see Alcatraz, Angel Island, the Golden Gate Bridge, and Marin (if it isn't foggy). If you look down you will see the original rocky shoreline.

- Continue through the Meadow to Laguna and Gashouse Cove to your beginning.

Further Ambling

If you wish, you can follow the Promenade along the water, in the direction of Fillmore (west) to the Marina Green. There you can see the people flying kites, and along the waterfront you can see coots, western grebes, and mallards. Mallow, oxalis, and tower of jewels bloom beside the walkway.

Walk Forward

Pacific Heights

But Always Look Back

When the first cable car went over Nob Hill in
1878, the development of Pacific Heights, the ridge
across the Polk-Van Ness Valley, soon followed. Then
as now, the views of the Bay were extraordinary.
Although a precipitous 370 feet above sea level, the
Heights had many wide, flat lots for the large homes only the
wealthy could afford.

The variety of architectural styles range from Italianates of the
late 1870s, elaborate Queen Anne Victorians of the 1890s, Mission
Revival, Edwardian, Italian Renaissance, to mock Chateau. Pacific
Heights is an excellent area to practice sightings of architectural
details—general, singular, and humorous.

◢ Begin at Broadway and Baker. Bliss and Faville, famous for
their designs of classical government buildings, built No. 2898
Broadway, on the northeast corner, in 1889. (A few blocks away on
Broadway, toward the end of this walk, you will see another Bliss
and Faville structure to compare.)

◢ Descend the two-block-long Baker Stairway. Monterey pines and
cypresses in the center area and dense shrubs on both sides confine
the stairway. In addition, the tread to riser proportion of the stairs
is not felicitous.

◢ Enter Vallejo. The large home on your left at No. 2901 Vallejo, built
in 1886, is a combination of Mediterranean and Mission styles. Turn

right to look at Nos. 2881 and 2891, which have extremely narrow second-story windows. These homes were originally connected and were modeled after a church.

◢ Continue on Baker to descend the lower section of the stairway on the right, which feels lighter and more cheerful than the upper section. Open space around the comfortable stairs makes this a happy, bouncy descent. No. 2511 is a redwood-shingled box with a twin-gabled roof.

There is no orthodoxy in walking. It is a land of many paths and no paths, where everyone goes his own way and is right.
—Dr. Trevelyan

◢ The Palace of Fine Arts is in the center of view, surrounded by the North Bay and the circle of hills beyond it. Similar houses at Nos. 2872 and 2880 Green that I find particularly appealing are to our left. Go to the end of the Green St. cul-de-sac to look at the variety and the unity of the architecture and the crown jewel at No. 2601 Lyon.

◢ Come back to the corner of Baker and continue walking along Green to Pierce. No. 2790 is the Russian Consulate. No. 2452 is a "tuck-in"; No. 2423 was built in 1891 by the architect Ernest Coxhead, who built his own house next door at No. 2421. No. 2411 has a slate roof.

◢ Turn right on Pierce to No. 2727 Pierce, an original farm mansion built in 1865 by Henry Casebolt. He was a blacksmith, builder, and inventor. He started the Sutter St. Railway (a horse car line) and invented the balloon car, an early form of the streetcar that was rounded and carried its own turntable. Continue to Broadway.

◢ Turn left on Broadway to Fillmore. Descend the Fillmore Stairway on the right side from Broadway to Vallejo. There are spectacular views from the west to the north. Continue descending the stairway from Vallejo to Green. Feel the difference in walking comfort between the stairway on the left, an L-shaped tread, and the one on the right, a sloping tread. No. 2323 Vallejo is the Vedanta Society Temple designed by Henry Gutterson and completed in 1959. The architecture is more subdued than the 1905 original temple on Filbert and Webster. Both temples are still in use. The basic philosophic tenet of Vedantism is that all paths to God are equally true. Everything comes from the divine spirit, and the purpose of life is to discover that unfolding spirit within us and everywhere else. Nearby are the monastery and convent, where men and women train to become monastics.

◢ Turn right on Green to Webster. No. 2160 Webster, built in 1867 for Leander Sherman of Sherman Clay music stores, has landmark status. Frequent musical evenings were hosted here. Visiting artists performed, among them Madame Ernestine Schumann-Heink and Ignace Jan Paderewski.

◢ Turn right on Webster to Vallejo and ascend the stairway to Broadway. At the top look back to see one of San Francisco's many views. Nos. 2120 and 2222 Broadway are two estates that belonged to the Flood family (of Comstock mine fortune) and are now private schools. The former, built in 1898 for James C. Flood, is the Sarah Dix Hamlin School for Girls. The gardens and tennis courts extend the depth of the lot to No. 2129 Vallejo, where an addition to the school was built in 1965; the two buildings are connected by a stairway. No. 2222 Broadway, the Convent of the Sacred Heart High School, was designed in 1912 for James L. Flood's son, J. C. This Italian Renaissance-style mansion by Bliss and Faville has an exterior of Tennessee marble; the interior has hand-carved wood

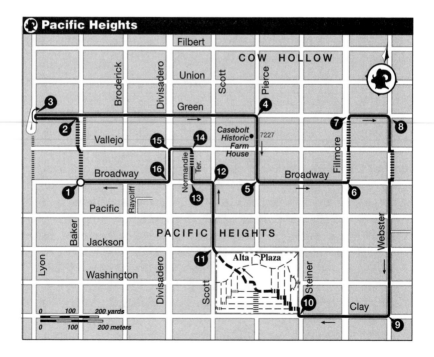

paneling of oak, satinwood, and walnut. (I'm sure the Hebrew tradition of placing honey on the first page of the first book a child reads, to promote sweet associations with learning, applies as well to learning in such beautiful surroundings.)

◢ Though it displays the pineapple finial, a symbol for hospitality, No. 2550 Webster is a heavy looking, uninviting, clinker-brick structure. Willis Polk built it in 1896 for William Bourn, who at various times was head of the Spring Valley Water Company, Pacific Gas and Electric, and the Empire Mining Company in Grass Valley. Polk also designed Filoli, Bourn's garden estate in Woodside, now part of the National Trust for Historic Preservation.

◢ The Newcomer High School formerly at Jackson and Webster has moved to 1350 7th Ave. It provides bilingual classes for almost 90 languages and transitional education for recently arrived immigrant students.

◢ At Nos. 2321–2315 Webster, between Jackson and Washington, are a series of slanted-bay Italianates that date from 1878. Calla lilies

---

WALK 7 ROUTE: Pacific Heights

Public Transportation: MUNI Bus #3 Jackson, #45 Union. For MUNI bus information, call 311 (outside San Francisco call (415) 701-2311).

1. Begin at Baker and Broadway. Descend two-block-long Baker Stwy. to Green.
2. Left on Green to view cul-de-sac.
3. Return on Green to Pierce.
4. Right on Pierce to Broadway.
5. Left on Broadway to Fillmore.
6. Left on Fillmore. Descend Fillmore (sidewalk) Stwy. on right to Green.
7. Right on Green to Webster.
8. Right on Webster. Ascend Webster (sidewalk) Stwy. at Vallejo. Continue to Clay.
9. Right on Clay to Steiner.
10. Ascend the Clay Stwy. of Alta Plaza Park. Walk across in a westerly direction to Jackson and Scott.
11. Right on Scott to Broadway.
12. Left on Broadway for a half block to Normandie Ter.
13. Walk to the end of the cul-de-sac. Descend stairway to Vallejo.
14. Left on Vallejo to Divisadero.
15. Left on Divisadero to Broadway.
16. Right on Broadway to Baker to your beginning.

and roses growing in the gardens complement the simple character of the houses. In the next block, between Washington and Clay, is a series of attached, slanted-bay Italianates, Nos. 2253–2233. These homes are in the Webster Historic District. Yet another group of Italianates, Nos. 2221–2209, round out the picture of the Victorian community. The California Pacific Medical Center, which presently dominates the area, has evolved from a merger of the University of Pacific Medical School and Presbyterian Hospital.

◢ Turn right on Clay. One block ahead to the right is No. 2318 Fillmore, the site of a stagecoach stop, now the Smith-Kettlewell Eye Research Institute.

◢ At Steiner you walk up the Clay Stairway of Alta Plaza Park, which was purchased in 1877. John McLaren, the superintendent of Golden Gate Park for 60 years, designed the 12 acres of excessively steep Alta Plaza in the only way possible—with slopes and terraces. The stairways are magnificent and the views varied. Looking down from the hill on the row of Italianates on Clay (Nos. 2637–2673), you appreciate the presence and the scale of these post–Civil War structures with their imposing false fronts.

◢ Walk across the park in a westerly direction toward Jackson and Scott; continue north on Scott to Broadway. Turn left on Broadway and right into Normandie Terrace, a special enclave of a few custom-designed homes. At the end of the cul-de-sac, descend the stairway. Turn left on Vallejo and left on Divisadero. At Broadway is another view to the east-northeast. Turn right on Broadway, but not before you find the sculpture *Goliath the Robot*, and then continue to Baker to your beginning.

Alta Plaza Park *Polly Gates*

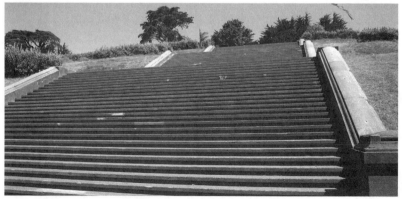

Tripping

Presidio Wall & Marina Waterfront—East & West

Lightly

On this walk you will trip lightly through
adjoining sections of three neighborhoods—Pacific
Heights, Letterman Digital Arts Center (George
Lucas's film campus), and lower sections of the Marina.
You'll experience a contrast in topography, from 379 feet to
sea level, and have the comfortable feeling that the neighborhoods fit together after all. Imagine you're on a vacation stroll.
Better yet, you're on an everyday stroll that is alive with beautiful
sights for the eyes.

The Presidio, the Marina harbor, the Palace of Fine Arts with its
surrounding lagoon and paths area, and Crissy Field's promenade and
beaches are magnets attracting people from everywhere out to enjoy
a day in the City. This area is part of the landfill site of the spectacular
Panama-Pacific International Exposition of 1915, celebrating the rebirth
of San Francisco after the 1906 earthquake. This extravagant and
most classic of fairs signaled all the world that San Francisco, like the
mythical phoenix, had arisen from the ashes of the 1906 earthquake to
become again the City that everybody loves.

◀ Begin your walk at the intersection of Lyon and Gorgas at the
Presidio Wall. Turn left on Gorgas. Walk on the sidewalk between
the two concrete columns, approximately seven feet high. Opposite
the four short green posts, turn left and walk through two handsome stone pillars to enter the unusual public garden designed

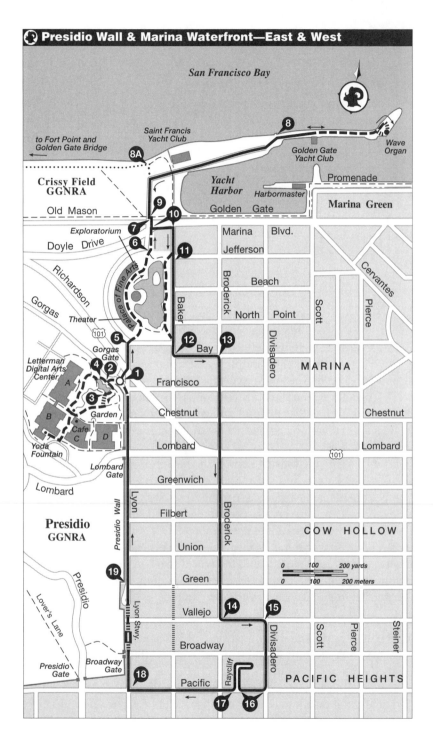

Presidio Wall & Marina Waterfront—East & West

San Francisco Bay

to Fort Point and
Golden Gate Bridge

Saint Francis
Yacht Club

8A

8

Golden Gate
Yacht Club

Wave
Organ

Crissy Field
GGNRA

Promenade

Yacht
Harbor

Harbormaster

Marina Green

Old Mason

Golden Gate

9

10

Exploratorium

Marina   Blvd.

Doyle Drive

Jefferson

7

6

Richardson

11

Beach

Cervantes

Gorgas

North   Point

Broderick

Scott

Pierce

Baker

Theater

5

Divisadero

12   Bay   **13**

Gorgas
Gate

Letterman
Digital Arts
Center

4 **2**

1

Francisco

MARINA

A

3

Chestnut

Chestnut

Garden

B

Cafe

Lombard

Lombard

C   D

Yoda
Fountain

Lombard
Gate

Greenwich

Lombard

**Presidio
GGNRA**

Presidio Wall

Lyon

Filbert

Broderick

COW HOLLOW

Union

Presidio

Green

0   100   200 yards

0   100   200 meters

19

Lover's Lane

Lyon Stwy.

Vallejo

14

15

Scott

Pierce

Steiner

Broadway

Divisadero

Presidio
Gate

Broadway
Gate

18

Pacific

Raycliff

PACIFIC HEIGHTS

17   **16**

by Lawrence Halprin Associates. This entrance is Gorgas Gate, unmarked at present.

◢ Ascend the stone stairway on the left and walk under a series of standing metal arches, embellished with cut steel maple leaves. The sun was shining and magnified reflections of the patterns were displayed on the sidewalks. The sight that caught my attention

---

WALK 8 ROUTE: Presidio Wall & Marina Waterfront— East & West

Public Transportation: MUNI Bus #28 19th Ave., #43 Masonic, #30 Stockton. For MUNI bus information, call 311 (outside San Francisco call (415) 701-2311).

1. Begin your walk at the turn of the Presidio Wall on Lyon. Turn left on Gorgas. Left at four green posts into Letterman Digital Arts Center garden (unmarked Gorgas Gate).
2. Left and ascend stone stairway. Walk past metal arches by the pond.
3. Ascend the stone slab stairway and walk the paths, see the sculptures, explore the area, and return to the Gorgas Gate.
4. Descend stairway to Gorgas at Lyon. Turn right to the crosswalks.
5. Follow the crosswalks to the Palace of Fine Arts. Walk into the inner courtyard and rotunda, strolling among the ruins. Continue to the Exploratorium.
6. At the Exploratorium front parking area, bear right to the crosswalk on Marina Blvd.
7. Walk across and continue to the water. Right toward the St. Francis Yacht Club.
8. Continue to the Golden Gate Yacht Club and the jetty's end to the Wave Organ. Return to the Crissy Field entrance.
8A. *Optional:* Walk west along the water on the Coastal Trail into Crissy Field to Fort Point and the Golden Gate Bridge. Return to Crissy Field entrance.
9. Walk back to Marina Blvd. and Lyon. Cross the boulevard.
10. Left to Baker, and right on Baker.
11. Walk along the front of the Palace of Fine Arts and lagoon to Bay.
12. Left on Bay to Broderick.
13. Right on Broderick to Vallejo.
14. Left on Vallejo to Divisadero.
15. Right on Divisadero to Pacific.
16. Right on Pacific to Raycliff Ter. Walk into cul-de-sac. Return to Pacific.
17. Right on Pacific to Lyon.
18. Right on Lyon. Descend Lyon Stwy.
19. Continue on Lyon to the end of the Presidio Wall to your beginning.

---

immediately was the abundance of field rocks and boulders and their placement—on low walls, alongside the falls, as well as around the lagoon. They come from the Redding, California, area. The garden imparts a sense of "There is time. You don't have to rush." I'm sure much of it comes from the rocks.

◢ Ascend the stone slab stairway to the path. At your own pace and direction, follow the paths and areas leading to a cafe and restaurant open to the public and four sculptures by Lawrence Noble: Eadweard Muybridge, the photographer famous for his experiment proving that all four legs of horses are off the ground at one point when running; Philo Farnsworth, inventor of television; Yoda at Bldg. B; and Willis O'Brien, animator of the original *King Kong* movie and stop-motion genius, in Bldg. B (open on weekdays only).

◢ George Lucas was awarded the privilege of leasing land for his film campus, Letterman Digital Arts Center (LDAC), which is, at this time, the largest leasee in the Presidio. Currently, the LDAC houses the Industrial Light and Magic and Lucas Arts. The employees number around 1,300. Skywalker Sound, another branch, is situated in Marin.

◢ The LDAC was in process for five years from the design stage to the opening. The architects were Gensler Architecture & Design and HKS, Inc. It is on the site of the dismantled Letterman Army Hospital, from which 80 percent of the materials—cement, metals, and timber—were recycled and used in the LDAC's construction. The archaeology is so recent that it is still easy for me to visualize the area as it was.

◢ The Gen II Otis elevators in the buildings are the most efficient in use of energy. Raised flooring allows for ventilation in all the buildings. The windows are designed for the best circulation of air. The center stairwells are sunlit to encourage people to use the stairs. Many aspects of the buildings encourage conservation of energy. In addition the LDAC bought new materials from suppliers within a short radius of the Presidio to cut down on travel and fuel. For all of these reasons, the campus received a LEED-gold certified rating from the Green Building Institute in 2006.

◢ Return to the Gorgas Gate, where you entered. A plaque on the top of the stairway states THIS SITE IS MANAGED AND MAINTAINED BY LETTERMAN DIGITAL ARTS LTD. Descend the stairway to Gorgas near Lyon. Veer to the right and follow the crosswalks to your left, across Richardson, to the Palace of Fine Arts. At Bay, walk on the path into the inner courtyard and rotunda. Bernard Maybeck designed the Palace of Fine Arts, the only architectural survivor of the 1915 Panama-Pacific International Exposition. The building has been renovated by the funds raised through the Maybeck Foundation, the City of San Francisco, and private sources.

◢ Bear left around the theater to the Exploratorium, a museum of science, art, and human perception (open Tuesday–Sunday 10 AM to 5 PM). Children and adults are encouraged to participate in the various exhibits by touching, looking, listening, and moving. High school students in the explainer program are available to answer questions. The Exploratorium was the idea of the late physicist and founding director Dr. Frank Oppenheimer and his wife, Jackie. One of the most vital museums in the City and a model for science museums throughout the world, the Exploratorium is scheduled to move to its new home, Piers 15 and 17, in 2013.

◢ At the Exploratorium's front parking area, walk to the crosswalk at Marina Blvd. Cross the street and continue to the water. Turn right toward the St. Francis Yacht Club. At the end of the parking lot is an impressive Rolex Clock. Continue to the Golden Gate Yacht Club to reach the Wave Organ at the jetty's end. This wave-activated acoustic sculpture was designed by Peter Richards, and built by sculptor and master stonemason George Gonzalez, under the aegis of the Exploratorium. It is situated in the sound garden the artists designed, a terraced amphitheater built of recycled marble and granite acquired from a dismantled cemetery. The idea was to sit, enjoy the view of the skyline, and listen to the water music as the pipes, which extend down into the Bay, respond to the movement of the water. The project was completed in spring of 1986, as part of the Exploratorium's science and art collection, and was dedicated to Frank Oppenheimer.

◢ Return to the Crissy Field entrance. As an optional side trip, you may continue along the water onto the Coastal Trail to reach the restored Crissy Field, a 20-acre tidal marsh with a new shoreline promenade and restored beach and dunes. Here you can observe the windsurfers and may even catch one of the regular windsurfing competitions. (Prior to 1915, Crissy Field was used as a dump by the Army; in the 1920s the space was used for an airfield and a rifle range.) You can continue on the trail to Fort Point, built in 1861 for defense against the South during the Civil War. Its walls are 7 feet thick and 45 feet high. It survived the 1906 earthquake. Retrace your steps to the Crissy Field entrance.

Edward Payson Weston began a 500-mile walk from San Francisco to Los Angeles on May 25, 1908. People were invited to join him at any point and walk as far as they wanted. He left the Olympic Club on Post St. at 12 PM sharp and reached Los Angeles in 10 days.

◢ Turn right and walk back to the Marina Blvd. Cross the boulevard at the crosswalk and turn left to Baker. At Baker turn right, walking along the front of the Palace of Fine Arts and the lagoon. The area around the lagoon is a popular place for people to picnic, sunbathe, and have their wedding parties photographed. In and around the lagoon, you will see swans, mallards, and night herons. When I was there, I identified a European widgeon, a bufflehead, and some coots. Turtles may be out on a sunny day, and sometimes you can see fish in the water.

◢ Turn left on Bay. Two murals in the 2300 block add a personal touch to the long block. Continue to Broderick, and then right on Broderick to walk uphill to Vallejo. The houses are eclectic and architecturally sound. No. 2821 Broderick and the house to the right were the earliest on the block, dating from about 1907.

◢ The sidewalk on Broderick from Vallejo to Broadway is extremely steep and uncomfortable to climb, plus it is private property—bypass it. Instead turn left on Vallejo to Divisadero. Turn right on Divisadero to Broadway. At Broadway look left for a spectacular view of the City's downtown. Continue to Pacific and turn right.

Lyon Stairway *Adah Bakalinsky*

- At Pacific walk into Raycliff Terrace, a cul-de-sac of six houses designed by contemporary architects.

- Return to Pacific and turn right and walk to Lyon. The El Drisco Hotel at 2901 Pacific (48 rooms) was built as a boardinghouse in 1903; it became a hotel in the 1930s. No. 2950 is a "tuck-in," inset some distance from the sidewalk. An unusual variance gives three houses at No. 3070 one driveway with entrances on both Pacific and Lyon.

- At the intersection of Pacific and Lyon you are 379 feet above sea level. This corner was named Cannon Hill for the symbolic cannon placed on the summit to mark the southeast corner of the Presidio (in the late 1870s). Turn right on Lyon to walk north along the Presidio Wall, enjoying a view of the Palace of Fine Arts's Romanesque rotunda, with the Marin hills as a backdrop.

- At Broadway descend the imposing Lyon Stairway—designed by Louis Upton in 1916—an arrangement of stairs, landings, and garden spaces. The Broadway neighbor to the right of the stairway has taken the initiative to renovate the gardens. The slope is covered with ivy. Surprisingly, it has a beautiful, undulating effect as you walk on the stairs. In spring, the blossoms on the plum trees and the colors and shapes of the annuals planted alongside the stairs draw you to them.

- On the ledge of the next set of stairs is a plaque dedicated to the memory of Ann Fogelberg, who spearheaded the Lyon St. Pride Project—the street cleanup and planting of trees and thousands of Vinca major plants on the slopes of Lyon Stairway between Vallejo and Green. She recruited neighborhood people, high school students, the Department of Public Works Environmental Street Services, and San Francisco Beautiful, as well as many others.

- The stairway ends in the cul-de-sac of Green. The six houses to your left, designed by architect August Headman and built in 1923, stand on part of the Miranda land grant, given to Corporal A. Miranda of the Presidio. Under the oval center is the Agua de Figueroa spring, where the Presidio horses quenched their thirst, as do the successfully growing three redwoods and cypress trees.

- Continue on Lyon, past Lombard (looking back occasionally to view the homes on the heights) to the end of the Presidio Wall to your beginning.

Further Ambling

Chestnut St., the Marina's authentic and stable shopping area, is again thriving after the effects of the devastating 1989 earthquake. It's fun to be part of the ambling, strolling shoppers and greet friends one hasn't seen since last week.

A Magical

Fort Winfield Scott—The Presidio

Walk

Presidio: (from Spanish) military post or fortified settlement

We are fortunate, living in San Francisco, to enjoy within the City boundaries a legacy of 1,490 acres of open space, which was home to the Native American Ohlone tribelet as far back as 3,000 years ago. Subsequently, the area became a Spanish military post (1776), a Mexican military post (1821), and then an American military post (1846–1994). In 1972, in one of its finest moments, Congress passed legislation creating the Golden Gate National Recreation Area (GGNRA). California Congressman Phillip Burton wrote this extraordinary law.

One of the stipulations of the GGNRA was that the Presidio, a U.S. Army post, would become part of the National Park Service and the GGNRA, if it was not needed by the Army. The Department of the Interior, in 1982, designated the Presidio as a National Historic Landmark and officially recognized 500 historic buildings. In the fall of 1994, the transfer went into effect.

Because the Presidio is so vast, has approximately 800 buildings, and will eventually have more than 50 miles of trails and eight scenic overlooks available for visitors to enjoy, the cost of maintaining such a wealth of natural and human-made resources is high. Therefore, in 1996, Congress created a new federal agency, the Presidio Trust to manage the noncoastal areas of the Presidio (1,192 acres). The Presidio Trust supervises and leases the residential and commercial properties with an objective of achieving financial self-sufficiency by 2013. From then on, income must meet expenses. Meanwhile, much good work is being done to promote the historical preservation and the natural

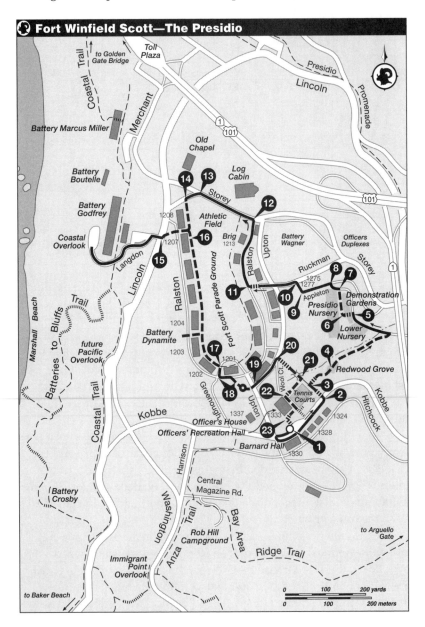

Fort Winfield Scott—The Presidio

Walk 9 ROUTE: Fort Winfield Scott—The Presidio

Public Transportation: MUNI Bus #28 19th Ave., #29 Sunset. Free PresidiGo Shuttle. For MUNI bus information, call 311 (outside San Francisco call (415) 701-2311). For PresidiGo Shuttle information, call (415) 561-5300.

Parking: Park in the lot across from Barnard Hall, 1330 Kobbe.

1. Cross Kobbe at the corner of Upton. Turn left toward No. 1324. Cross Kobbe at the crosswalk.

2. Descend stairway, and continue ahead on walkway.

3. Right to descend second set of stairs. Continue to the open space.

4. Walk to the right through the redwood grove and down right side of seasonal creek to the lower area of Presidio Nursery and demonstration gardens on hillsides. Turn left.

5. Bear left to ascend peeler-core stairway to the upper portion of the Presidio Nursery.

6. Right past greenhouses.

7. Left between buildings and parking area.

8. Left on Appleton at No 1275.

9. Right at No. 1277 to Ruckman.

10. Left on Ruckman and walk on left side. Ascend the sidewalk stairways to Ralston.

11. Right on Ralston past the Brig to Storey.

12. Left on Storey (detour to look at Log Cabin across the street). Continue on Storey.

13. Bear left on the first street (around baseball field) to No. 1208.

14. Left at No. 1208 onto the Ft. Scott Walkway.

15. Right between Nos. 1208 and 1207 and cross Lincoln Blvd. at Langdon Court. Follow Bay Area Ridge Trail sign to Battery Godfrey. Explore and return to No. 1208.

16. Right at No. 1207, following the Ridge Trail to No. 1204. Turn right to walk between Nos. 1204 and 1203 to look at Battery Dynamite. Explore and return to No. 1203. Continue to No. 1202.

17. Right to Ralston.

18. Left on Ralston and walk on an old concrete path that crosses the lawn at the corner of Ralston and Upton.

19. Continue straight ahead then downhill on Upton to the intersection of Upton and Wool Court.

20. At the intersection street sign, descend stone stairways, cross bridge, ascend stairway.

21. Right at first path. Walk along tennis court, up to a paved parking area.

22. Left and walk alongside the curved window wall of the Officers' Recreation Hall, No. 1333.

23. Then right, at end of the building, to ascend the curved stairway to the parking lot across from No. 1330 Kobbe, to your beginning.

diversity of the area. Some of the projects include developing habitat to increase the population of 200 species of birds year-round, including migratory and resident varieties; replacing eucalyptus trees that have reached their 100-year maturity with native trees; and restoring Lobos Creek, the water source for the Presidio. I personally am delighted by the dedication of the staff and volunteers and the direction the Presidio is taking in working with open space, views, and native plant areas. There are 1,109 units available for housing. The housing is leased at market prices except for a few accommodations for resident rangers and park police. Some units have been set aside for low-cost housing. I begin a walk as a stroll. I don't know what I'm looking for, but suddenly, something appeals to me. In this case it's a series of river-washed rocks fashioned into very long, low retaining walls along Kobbe Ave., the street lined with officers' homes. Then I discover river-rock wall supports along stairways leading to woodsy paths among random rows of eucalyptus trees and Monterey pines. As I walk down the stairways and step into leafy, overgrown areas that continue for a distance, the atmosphere changes. It has a primeval quality and a feeling of mystery. I am eager to continue.

I am in the western section of the Presidio, known as Fort Winfield Scott. In 1912, the Coast Artillery Group was formed to protect the coast. It was and still is part of the Presidio, but it was given its own fort, named after the general. I parked in the nearby lot, but I encourage you to use the free PresidiGo Park Shuttles. As of this printing, PresidiGo runs every 30 minutes seven days a week (6:30 AM–7:30 PM Monday–Friday and 11 AM–6 PM Saturday, Sunday, and holidays). Obtain current schedules at www.presidio.gov; call the Trust Transportation Department at (415) 561-5300; or pick up a free PresidiGo schedule and map of the area at the Presidio Visitors' Center in the Old Officers club at No. 50 Moraga (the entrance is notable for a nearby cannon). You can also call (415) 561-4323 and request that the information be mailed to you. I unequivocally recommend taking the circle tour to become familiar with the general layout of the park.

◢ Park across the street from Barnard Hall, 1330 Kobbe St., the building known as BOQ—Bachelor Officers' Quarters. The residences along this street were formerly used for officers and their families. At the Upton intersection cross Kobbe. Walk left to No. 1324 (three houses down), built in 1912. In 1883 Major William A. Jones submitted a plan for introducing trees to the Presidio. Acacia, pine, eucalyptus, native redwood, madrone, spruce, and palm were planted in the 1880s and 1890s, many of them by schoolchildren on Arbor Day. Cross Kobbe at the crosswalk, opposite No. 1324. Descend the concrete stairway with sidewalls of river rock. Part of the walkway is brick.

◢ After many years of neglect, the forest is being rehabilitated. Each time I walk here the setting has changed from an overgrown, wild mass of ivy and mattress wire weed (Muehlenbeckia) and broken and dying trees to an area providing optimum conditions for happy, healthy trees and shrubs to grow and to provide home and food for birds and wildlife. Continue down the stairs and next to the tennis courts turn right to descend another small set of stairs to a footpath that leads, a few feet farther on, to open space. (There are six tennis courts in various places throughout the Presidio, all managed by the Presidio YMCA.)

◢ Continue toward the right, through a redwood grove, downward on the footpath, which is considered a "social" trail because it was created by walkers and not the Park Service. Follow along the right side of Dragonfly Creek, which, though always damp, is relatively dry in September and wet in the winter. Farther on, past the nursery, it is culverted to Crissy Field. On your left, lying helter-skelter on the ground, is a collection of granite slabs with incised names, rubble left from the 1906 earthquake. These historic slabs were originally stored at Lands End, but brought to the Presidio because people were removing them for their personal collections. In front of you is the lower section of the Presidio Nursery, shade houses that are open and allow temperate climate control. The Park Conservancy, a nonprofit group, manages the test planting and restoration work with a staff of two full-time horticulturalists, as well as interns and volunteers. Participants are welcome to assist on Wednesdays and Saturdays from 1 PM to 4 PM. The Presidio nursery is the largest nursery in the entire GGNRA; seedlings for Crissy Field are grown here.

◢ Turn left to note the flagged demonstration garden along the hillside on both sides. The demonstration garden showcases the various habitats that occur in the Presidio, from oak woodland to sandy dunes to serpentine grassland. Turn left at the small bridge and ascend the peeler-core stairway to the upper Presidio Nursery. The nursery is clean of debris and so well organized, with containers of young plants in alphabetic order, ready to be dispersed according to plan, I feel I could come in for the first time and know where to find what I needed. The nursery area is undergoing renovation but, during this time, the Habitarium will continue to function.

⬛ Children five years or older, as well as adults, are welcome and encouraged to participate in the Presidio Nursery program, which is part of the curriculum for grades six through eight. Summer camp is also available. I'm told that one of the favorite activities of the junior high and high school students is planting in the rain, when the soil is at optimum consistency and the process feels like fingerpainting, on a grand scale. A permanent Center for Sustainability, which will contain classrooms, lab rooms, and kitchen and bathroom facilities and will accommodate larger numbers of students and adults, is scheduled to be built nearby.

⬛ To the right of the stairway there are greenhouses with native plant seedlings grown under optimum conditions. Walk past the greenhouses and veer left between the buildings and parking lot. Walk to the unmarked street, Appleton. You will see the sign No. 1275 across the street. Turn left and walk past the row of enlisted-family housing on the right that has been renovated for leasing. A view of downtown San Francisco is behind you.

⬛ Turn right at No. 1277 to Ruckman, then left. Walk on the left side, pass Upton, and ascend short sidewalk stairways to Ralston. Turn right and pass the Brig, a flat-roofed, two-story building. You might think that the Brig once offered its inmates the best views. It would have if the windows were at eye level, but the second-story floor is so low that one needs a ladder to see out of the window. Many windows on the other buildings have bars across them, which were added for protection in case someone accidentally forgot to close the windows.

⬛ Continue on Ralston to Storey. The Log Cabin is straight ahead. It was built of timber logs and rock in 1937 by the Works Progress Administration. The interior has wagon wheel chandeliers, a huge fireplace, space for large groups to dine or dance, and a view of the meadow and San Francisco. For rental information, call (415) 561-5444. Go left on Storey, then bear left on the first street around the softball field to No. 1208. Turn left at 1208 to continue on the Fort Scott Walkway. Turn right between Nos. 1208 and 1207.

⬛ Cross Lincoln Blvd. at the Langdon Court crosswalk, to follow a small section of the Bay Area Ridge Trail. (Watch for cars.) Follow the trail sign to Battery Godfrey and explore the area a bit. An interpretive sign gives some of its history. One very clear day I looked out and saw the Farallon Islands—a historic moment! The norm is overcast, hidden islands. From this viewpoint, you see the curved Golden Gate Bridge span. I've walked across the bridge; I've driven across the Bridge. I never felt the curve. This view adds another dimension to my friendship with the bridge. (For more bridge view locations, see Further Ambling on page 86.)

◢ Return to the Fort Scott Walkway. Cross Lincoln Blvd. at the crosswalk. At the side of No. 1208, looking toward the green meadow, you see the Bay Bridge, which I call the Cinderella Bridge—by day, it is a working bridge; by night, it becomes a sparkling phantom bridge, enveloped by glittering lights. (A friend suggested the "Two Bridge Walk" as a title.) You also see Coit Tower and Russian Hill. Continue walking alongside the enlisted men's barracks, which are built of concrete and stucco, in the Mission Revival–style. Italian stone pines, which reach maturity after 50 to 70 years, have been planted along the row. The pine in front of No. 1206 is striking, with its large galls surrounding the trunk. Galls are part of the tree, and not a disease, I was delighted to learn.

◢ Turn right to walk back between Nos. 1204 and 1203, and go into Battery Dynamite if the gate is open. What you see first is a 40-foot wall. There is a series of tunnels underneath, with three gun pits used for testing dynamite weapons during the 1890s.The problem of how to light the fuse without causing an explosion was solved by using the small, hidden Greek-style structure to the right of the wall as an air compressor for the new dynamite test guns, which operated like huge air compression rifles. The tests were successful. The shells could land in the water near a ship, and the concussion would break the hull. There was one problem: the short range of two miles. Since other coast-defense guns with a longer range were being developed, the dynamite test weapon was laid to rest.

"Well, here we go, up the apple and pears." This Cockney expression from east end of London means, "Here we go, up the stairs."

◢ Return to the Parade Ground and continue to No. 1202 to read the interpretive sign for Fort Winfield Scott. Turn right and continue to Ralston. Turn left and walk on the concrete path that crosses the lawn at the corner of Ralston and Upton. The area must have been a garden at some earlier time.

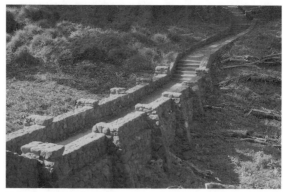

Upton at Wool Court   *Tony Holiday*

⊿ Continue straight ahead, down Upton to the intersection of Wool
   Court and Upton. At the intersection street sign, descend the stone
   stairways and walk across the stone bridge. The slopes have been
   cleared and planted. Along this trail I saw an Oregon junco and a
   spotted towhee. Continue to ascend stairway.

⊿ At the first path, turn right next to the tennis court. The mattress
   wire vine you may see is being gradually eradicated to prevent
   suffocation of other plants. Turn left alongside the curved window
   wall of the Officers' Recreation Hall, No. 1331. Turn right at the end
   of the building and ascend the curved stairway to your beginning.

Further Ambling

Opposite Battery Godfrey, at the tree line, a sign notes BAKER BEACH
AND BATTERIES TO BLUFFS TRAIL. This path leads to multiple stairways,
ascending and descending, along the bluffs of the Pacific Ocean to
Battery Chamberlain at Baker Beach. If you want to continue, cross
Lincoln Blvd. and ascend the connector stairway to Immigrant Point
Overlook and the Rob Hill Campground. You can return on the same
route or walk the Coastal Trail along Lincoln Blvd. back to Langdon.

Sutro's Legacy

Lands End

for All Time

Since my last visit to the Lands End area six
months ago, there have been welcome changes.
Thanks to the Richard and Rhoda Goldman Fund, for
their contribution of $2.6 million, plus $400,000 for a fea-
sibility study on renovating this Lands End landmark, we
now have graceful paved footpaths, new views of the bay,
new, comfortable redwood stairways, and attractively designed
direction signs. We have the opportunity of awaking our senses,
and taking in the colors and sounds of a wilderness area surrounded
by ocean and bay, and yet we are within the City.

From Point Lobos Ave. and El Camino del Mar, we are in an area of
the City known as the Sutro District, named for one of my favorite San
Francisco heroes, Adolph Sutro. The majority of wealthy citizens in the
late 1800s settled in the Nob Hill, Rincon Hill, and South Park neighborhoods. Sutro settled and developed the northwest part of the City,
which he loved for its beauty and fog and ocean air. As it evolved, he
understood its potential as open space and parkland and recreation to
be enjoyed by families.

Sutro came to the United States in 1850 from Aix La Chapelle with
his mother and seven siblings. He was 20 years old. He had a high
school education, worked in the family cloth factory, read voraciously,
and was self-taught in mining and engineering. He left us a profound
and beneficent legacy. Using the profits he accrued from the sale of
his shares in his first large engineering project in the United States,
the four-mile long tunnel built to drain and ventilate the Nevada

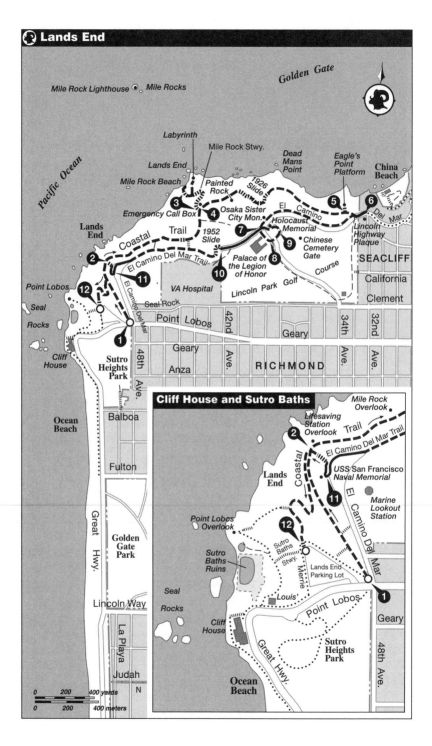

Comstock silver mines, Sutro developed and designed the Sutro Baths, an elaborate arrangement of pools with varying temperatures, to be enjoyed by families. He built the Sutro Railroad to provide low-cost (five cents) transportation for family outings—swimming in the Sutro Baths, dining at the Cliff House, or walking on the grounds of his 21-acre Sutro Heights Estate of sculpture and landscaped gardens.

Sutro planted trees to hold the soil of the sand dunes (while his choice of species was not appropriate for San Francisco, they held the soil, and the trees are gradually being replaced). He founded the Sutro Library and even opened his private property to the general public. He was mayor from 1894 to 1896 and died in 1898. Sutro Heights,

Walk 10 ROUTE: Lands End

Public Transportation: MUNI Bus #31 Balboa St., #38 Geary. For MUNI bus information, call 311 (outside San Francisco call (415) 701-2311).

1. Begin at El Camino Del Mar and Point Lobos Ave. at the Sutro District sign. Walk on the right paved footpath past stairways to the interpretive sign.
2. Continue veering right on the Coastal Trail. Pass the stairway leading to the USS *San Francisco* Naval Memorial, and continue past retaining walls. Descend a log stairway, and pass another stairway on the right. Turn left at the junction.
3. At the Mile Rock Beach sign, descend the Mile Rock Stwy. to the beach and Maze at Lands End.
4. Return to the Coastal Trail. Turn left and pass Painted Rock. Ascend the long stairway, and descend other shorter stairways.
5. At the stairways, Dead Man's Point is on your left. Continue to Eagle's Point Platform.
6. Continue on the Coastal Trail to El Camino Del Mar into Seacliff. Right on 32nd Ave. to view Lincoln Highway post.
7. Return to El Camino Del Mar (at 32nd Ave.) and continue on the right side of the road toward the Palace of the Legion of Honor and turn left.
8. Walk to the museum. Across the road at the bus stop is the Lincoln Highway plaque.
9. Walk past the pool to the *Holocaust Memorial*. Turn left to walk past the Osaka Sister City Monument.
10. Walk through the parking area. Descend the wood stairway to El Camino Del Mar Trail. It leads to a dirt path and boardwalk. Continue on the trail to the USS *San Francisco* Naval Memorial.
11. To the right of the memorial, descend the stairway to the Coastal Trail and turn left.
12. At a fork in the road, veer right. Continue toward the Merrie Way (Lands End) parking lot. Turn left and continue to your beginning.

Sutro Baths Ruins, and the Cliff House are now under the jurisdiction of the Golden Gate National Recreation Area.

◢ Begin your walk at El Camino Del Mar and Point Lobos Ave. at the Sutro District GGNRA sign. Walk on the right paved footpath to the Coastal Trail, 0.3 mile. Lawrence Halprin, the landscape architect whose work we will be viewing as we continue our walk, is well-known for his attention to greening within the context of the urban environment. The succulents and native plants that accompany our walk feel like the perfect solution for the setting. The plants are tended and planted by large groups of volunteers. (If you are interested in this work, call (415) 561-5333.) We find along the paths native plants, such as the sticky monkeyflower, lupines, and the California poppies. The multitude of yellow flowers, the little yellow sorrel on long stems, that abound along the footpaths are beautiful, but they are weeds and will take over an area. The National Parks Conservancy and National Park Service are doing their best to eradicate them. The Brush Sculpture, made from cut tree refuse is a haven for birds. We hear many white crown sparrows.

◢ Walk past the two stairways to the interpretive sign. Continue veering right and walk past the stairway leading to the USS *San Francisco* Naval Memorial.

◢ You may soon hear foghorns. Their sounds may be coming from the Golden Gate Bridge, Point Bonita Lighthouse, or Mile Rock (a mile from the middle of the shipping channel, not a mile from shore). Each foghorn has a recognizable pattern of timed seconds of sound followed by timed seconds of silence. From the right side of the trail you may periodically hear the gurgling sound of water, indicating a seep. Usually, you'll find a patch of green or flowers nearby, but watch out for the poison oak.

◢ As you continue on the Coastal Trail, you see a concrete wall on the right side. Built as the retaining wall for the Sutro Railroad, it continues to support the hillside. A landslide in 1925 closed off most of the rail lines. Shipwreck spotters liked to come here via the railroad, which came from Presidio Ave. and California along the cliffs. Most shipwrecks occurred through some combination of fog, northwest winds, sand bars, and rocky shoals. At low tide you can see remains of an engine block from the wreck of the *Lyman Stewart* and the sternpost of the *Frank Buck*. These can be viewed best at the next retaining walls and overlook. During World War II the Army

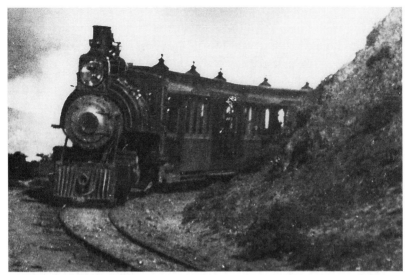

Sutro Railroad, ca. 1890 *Courtesy of National Park Service*

had coastal defenses and gun batteries along the cliff line here and spotting stations at Sutro Heights.

⊿ Continue on the unpaved footpath, descend a short log stairway, and pass a stairway on your right that leads to El Camino Del Mar Trail. This area has suffered landslides during heavy winter rains, and parts of the trail may be closed. Walk on any alternate path as indicated.

⊿ Walk past some serpentine and granite rocks. When the path ends, continue left to the MILE ROCK BEACH sign and stairway. The Mile Rock Stairway is well-built, comfortable to walk, and leads you to the ocean where waves continually crash against the huge rocks. Ascend the path to the right to see the Maze, constructed in the sand at the point of Lands End by Eduardo Aguilera. Walk it and solve it. The nude beaches are nearby. The return up the stairway is moderately difficult. If you prefer to omit this stairway, continue on the Coastal Trail. Painted Rock on your right was a Coast Guard navigational tool used as a sight line with Point Bonita Lighthouse in the Marin Headlands.

⊿ Just ahead in the fenced area on your left (a warning sign at Painted Rock cliff) was the tunnel through which Sutro's train rounded the bend. The tunnel collapsed, the cliff partially fell away, and the trail has been routed uphill—around to the right.

- Ascend the long stairway and curve left to descend shorter stairways. You will pass Dead Man's Point on the left, and then reach Eagle's Point Platform, which you can ascend via a ramp or stairway. As you walk across the platform, you have the opportunity to savor slightly varied views of Seacliff, China Beach, Baker Beach, the Golden Gate Bridge, and Fort Point. Return to the path.

- Turn left and walk to the end of the trail. Cross El Camino Del Mar, turn left to 32nd Ave. On the left side of 32nd Ave. is a commemorative post for the Lincoln Highway, the first transcontinental highway, which was built in 1915. It extended from Times Square in New York City to Lincoln Park in San Francisco. Retrace your steps and turn right into the Seacliff neighborhood. Seacliff was developed in 1924, with curving streets and gateway entrances at 25th, 26th, and 27th Aves. Homes are large, ocean views from north-facing windows are vivid, and gardens on the south side are verdant.

- Mark Daniels, former general superintendent and landscape engineer of the U.S. National Parks, laid out the system of curving streets and terraces. (He also designed the street pattern in Forest Hill, Walk 15.) The architect Willis Polk designed three homes in Seacliff—Nos. 9, 25, and 45 Scenic Way.

Post commemorating the Lincoln Highway

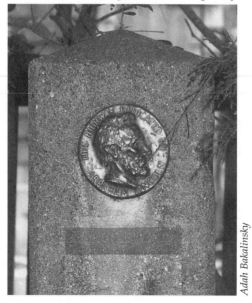

Adah Bakalinsky

◢ Recollecting his childhood, a former resident of Seacliff remembers walking through the sand dunes and the seas of gold and purple lupine. Rabbits, snakes, and wild canaries lived in the area then; he remembers his father trapping the canaries and feeding them hard-boiled eggs. He also recalls fishing every other day from Lands End.

◢ When you are ready to begin the return route, go back to El Camino Del Mar (at 32nd Ave.) and walk on the right side toward the Palace of the Legion of Honor. Continue walking past 17 memorial benches and the World Peace Monument along the way. Views of the Bay are to the right. The path borders the Lincoln Park Golf Course. At the *Holocaust Memorial*, turn left to the Palace of the Legion of Honor. If you wish to see the current exhibit and have lunch in the museum, go in (members get in free, but other visitors must pay an entry fee).

◢ On the knoll of the Lincoln Park Golf course are some of the remains of the 1868 cemetery. More than 1,000 graves, many of them Chinese, were discovered when the museum was retrofitted and redesigned in 1993. To see the one remaining Chinese cemetery gate, walk down the Legion of Honor Drive for about one-tenth of a mile. The gate will be on your left, in the middle of the golf course, easily seen embedded between two cypress trees. (Do not walk onto the golf course.)

◢ Across from the museum at the bus stop is a plaque that reads THIS HIGHWAY DEDICATED TO ABRAHAM LINCOLN. It's a replacement of the original one that disappeared. Three sides of the post display replicas of Lincoln's face.

◢ Walk toward the pool to see the outdoor sculptures: Closest to the pool is *Pax Jerusalem* by Mark di Suvero, a large orange abstract. *The Holocaust Memorial* by George Segal is to the left of the pool. To get the full emotional impact of the sculpture, view it from the platform. Toward the left is the Osaka Sister City Monument.

◢ Turn left beyond the monument along the paved parking area. Descend the wood stairway onto the El Camino Del Mar Trail. Continue walking on the path past the stairway to the Coastal Trail. The building seen above to your left is the VA Hospital.

◢ The path leads to the parking lot on El Camino Del Mar where the USS *San Francisco* Naval Memorial is located. The memorial was formed from the bridge of the ship after it was torpedoed in November 1942 during the Battle of Guadalcanal.

◢ In this area, there once existed a series of signal stations, where people were stationed to spot different ships coming in through the Golden Gate. They would then relay the information, originally via semaphores and later via telegraph, to the wharf area. One relay station structure, the Octagon House, remains above the parking lot, up toward the trees on the left. A semaphore attached to it was used to relay the particular ship's arrival to Telegraph Hill and Fisherman's Wharf. When electricity became available, the telegraph replaced the semaphores.

◢ Descend the stairway to the right of the memorial to the Coastal Trail, and turn left. At the fork in the road, veer right. Along the path is a continuation of the new native plantings of the coastal dunes. Before you reach the stairway into Merrie Way (Lands End) parking lot, turn left to your beginning.

Further Ambling

In the days when the Sutro Baths were operating, Adolph Sutro installed amusement rides where the Merrie Way (Lands End) parking lot is located. Interpretive signs are near the walkway. From there, descend the stairway to the Sutro Baths ruins. The baths were opened in 1896 and closed in 1952, and the buildings were destroyed by fire in 1966. In this eroded sandstone setting, with the offshore Seal Rocks in the background, are broken columns, fragments of tile mosaic, and the emptied pool area extending oceanward. The sea lions, formerly at home on Hermit Rock, moved to Pier 39 in 1989 for a reason that remains unknown. The sea lions may have moved as a result of the Loma Prieta earthquake or perhaps some other natural phenomenon. (As early explorers approached from the ocean side a distance away, Angel and Alcatraz islands looked like a continuous horizon line rather than islands in a bay. This explains why San Francisco was discovered via a land route from the south, rather than from the sea.)

In 1865 James Cooke walked from the Cliff House to Seal Rocks on a tightrope.

Bear right to the Point Lobos Overlook. The view of the Pacific Ocean and the Marin Headlands is mesmerizing. When you're ready to continue, walk on the curving path toward the right among the ruins. As you explore the area, please follow designated paths only.

You are allowed to enter the open tunnel that Sutro dug during the construction of the baths. The inside path can be slippery. To your left are the former pools, one of freshwater, the others salt. The honeycomb rectangle was the heating plant. Adolph Sutro designed and engineered the structure with its seven indoor pools, each heated to a different temperature. A swim, rental of a suit, towels, and locker cost $0.25. There was room for 10,000 swimmers and seats for 7,000 spectators. The conservatories were decorated with palm trees and Egyptian artifacts.

Return on the path and walk past the Sutro Baths Stairway. Primrose, lupine, poison oak, blackberry, and nasturtium grow alongside the path. You can also see dune tansy, blue bush lupine, beach primrose, and coyote bush. Park botanists are cultivating plants native to the area. Albizia, the tall shrub with white spiky flowers, grows everywhere. It's beautiful, but invasive.

Ascend the incline toward Louis' Restaurant on Point Lobos Ave. To the right is the remodeled Cliff House. In addition to the two restaurants you are welcome to view historical photos of Sutro Baths, Sutro Heights, and the Cliff House. If you want to explore the famous grounds of Sutro's home, walk to the arterial stop to cross Point Lobos Ave. This area is rich in all directions for exploring.

Another ambling jaunt takes you to the hiking paths along the Great Highway south of Balboa that have been tastefully landscaped for hikers and cyclists (sand control is more successful now than formerly).

If you would like to explore China Beach to the east, continue on El Camino Del Mar to Seacliff Ave. and China Beach. A stone has been placed at the top of the China Beach Stairway to commemorate the Chinese fishermen who used this site. If you would like to continue farther to Baker Beach, follow the sign at No. 320 El Camino Del Mar that says PUBLIC BEACH. Turn left on Seacliff, and at 25th Ave. turn left into the cul-de-sac to take the stairway to Baker Beach.

The MUNI Bus #29 and the PresidiGo Bus stop near Baker Beach. For a full-day's outing, continue on El Camino Del Mar to the Presidio, take Lincoln Blvd. to Fort Point, and continue on waterfront paths around Fisherman's Wharf and down the Embarcadero and the Blue Greenway (see Walks 6, 8, 9, and 29). With almost 4,000 acres of the GGNRA within the City, your walking opportunities are boundless!

Lead Thread

Golden Gate Heights

on a Sugar Sack

The vast tract of land known as the Sunset District sprawls south from Golden Gate Park to Sloat Blvd. and from Stanyan to the Pacific Ocean. At one time it was all sand dunes, and a Sunday's outing to the beach, with lunch or dinner at the Cliff House on the Great Highway, was a gala occasion. Silting is a continual problem, but it has been minimized on the Great Highway by a design of raised paths for bicyclists and pedestrians, plus the planting of dune tansy and ice plant. The Outer Sunset is subjected to magnificent sunsets, the ocean view, clean air, and wind and fog. The establishment of Golden Gate Park in 1870 promoted the settlement of the Sunset. Other events continued the process: A railroad was built along H Street (Lincoln Way) to the beach in 1879; in 1898 U.C. Medical School was established; in 1904 a Midwinter Fair was held in Golden Gate Park; and in 1905 St. Anne's Church was founded. The 1906 earthquake brought people to the outer lands, away from the damaged areas of Telegraph Hill, North Beach, and Russian Hill.

Mass housing techniques perfected in the 1920s were utilized by the three leading contractor/builders in the Sunset: Henry Doelger, Raymond Galli, and Fred Gellert. The new process enabled them to sell homes in the late 1930s for $5,000. Construction recommenced in 1945 after the end of World War II. Development of homes with tunnel entrances, the "Sunset look," where living rooms were built above garages, solved problems posed by smaller (25' x 65') lots and the low

$6,000 ceiling of available FHA loans. Between 60 and 80 percent of the homes are owner-occupied.

The Inner Sunset has a stable population of middle-class families of various ethnic origins. According to a 2008 report, Asians comprise 48.5%, Whites 44.9%, African Americans 1.33%, and Hispanics 4.5% (with the remaining 0.77% lumped into "Other").

Golden Gate Heights is one of the Sunset neighborhoods. Scouting the walk was reminiscent of trying to find the beginning loop thread on a 10-pound sugar sack. With one pull, I automatically unlock the other loops. When I found the lead stairway in Golden Gate Heights, all the other stairways "unlocked" and I felt as if I was on a Matisse walk—an uninterrupted rhythmic line with many curves.

◢ Begin the walk by ascending the mosaic tile stairway at 16th Ave. and Moraga. Children call it "the magic stairway." It is another of the fine examples of united community action that occurs in San Francisco. A young woman who lived in Rio de Janeiro and saw from her apartment window the Santa Teresa decorative stairway thought it would be wonderful if the concrete stairway she saw from her San Francisco window would sing with colors instead of nondescript grey. She began talking with neighbors, found a kindred spirit living next door to the stairway who wholeheartedly endorsed the project, and volunteered her garage (and her wonderful baking skills) for neighborhood meetings and presentations of possible stairway designs by artists. Discussions with City officials of plans and fees; talks with possible donors of tile, paints, and equipment; and consultations regarding fund-raising ideas and events ensued over a period of three years.

◢ People now come from afar to see and walk the stairway. Busloads of senior citizens, schoolchildren, and preschool tots and their parents—all are entranced by the colorful mosaic tile stairway that tells a story of sky and water and birds and fish and flowers and frogs. On August 27, 2005, the newly designed stairway by local mosaic artists, Colette Crutcher and Aileen Barr, was dedicated. The Lion Dancers performed, there were refreshments, the street was blocked off, the neighborhood was there, and Mayor Francesco Pignataro of Caltagirone, Italy, spoke eloquently. The famous Scala steps in his town was one source of inspiration for the 16th Ave. project. The citizens of this Italian town celebrate their stairway with an annual lighting of the stairs with hundreds of oil-filled cups called "coppi," that create astounding patterns of light.

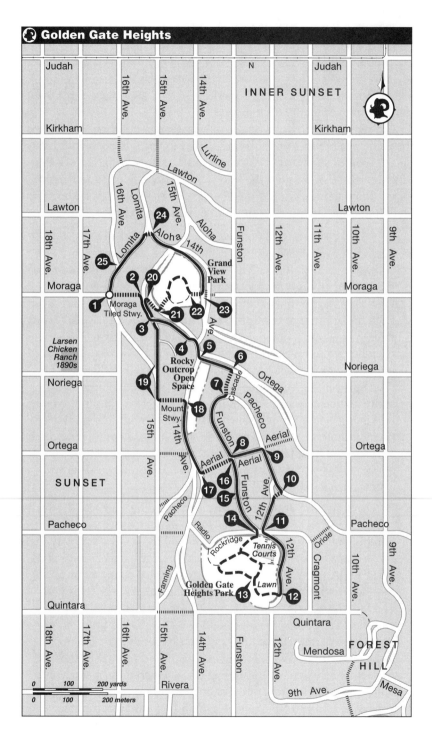

WALK 11 ROUTE: Golden Gate Heights

Public Transportation: MUNI Bus #66 Quintara; #28 19th Ave.; Metro N Judah. For MUNI bus or Metro information, call 311 (outside San Francisco call (415) 701-2311).

1. Begin at Moraga and 16th Ave. Ascend tiled stairway to 15th Ave.
2. Right on 15th Ave to Noriega.
3. Left on Noriega to 14th Ave.
4. Right on 14th Ave. to Ortega.
5. Left on upper Ortega to Cascade Stwy.
6. Right and ascend to intersection of Funston and Pacheco.
7. Right on Funston to Aerial.
8. Left on Aerial to Pacheco.
9. Right on Pacheco to the triangular piece of land at 12th Ave.
10. Ascend curved stairway to 12th Ave.
11. Left on 12th Ave. to intersection of Rockridge and Cragmont across from Golden Gate Heights Park.
12. Cross the street and turn left to walk on the sidewalk. At No. 2026 cross the street and enter park on paved path. Walk through playground and turn left.
13. Follow this path to the roundabout and sitting area at the top of the park. Continue on path around north side. Turn left at tennis courts and walk to Rockridge.
14. Cross Rockridge to Funston.
15. Continue on Funston to Aerial Stwy.
16. Descend Aerial Stwy. to 14th Ave.
17. Right on 14th Ave. to Mount Stwy.
18. Descend Mount Stwy. (next to No. 1795 14th Ave.) to 15th Ave.
19. Right on 15th Ave. past Noriega to stairway at retaining wall.
20. Ascend stairway. Cross upper 15th Ave.
21. Ascend stairway to Grand View Park.
22. Walk left on sand footpath at second bench around park. On opposite side of park, descend stairway to 14th Ave.
23. Left on 14th Ave. to intersection of 14th Ave., 15th Ave., and Aloha.
24. Veer left on Aloha to corner stairway onto Lomita.
25. Continue left on Lomita to 16th Ave. Veer left to your beginning.

I could see the tiled steps from the bus just before we stopped. I was amazed how brilliant the colors were even under such bad weather conditions. The overall design with changing patterns and colors were most impressive. As we approached the last tiers there were even some mirrors. I counted the steps in each tier and got a total of 162. With my altimeter watch I measured the total height at 100 feet.

—R. F., a walker from Southern California

◢ As you reach the fifth landing of the Moraga Stairway, glance to the left. The Golden Gate Bridge and its two towers should be visible. You will be alerted to shifts in optical illusion during the walk.

◢ At 15th Ave. turn right and walk to Noriega. Turn left and walk on the lower portion of Noriega. Turn right on 14th Ave. (near No. 1751) and bear left along the upper section of Ortega. The hill on the corner of Ortega and 14th Ave., also being restored by the Native Plant Society, is a large expanse of exposed Franciscan Formation outcropping. No. 601 Ortega (1953) is built on it. I think the house is one of the most dramatically sited residences in San Francisco. Two other houses were subsequently built on neighboring lots, mitigating the drama of the entire hill area.

◢ Turn right on Cascade Stairway, an unexpected "tuck-in" and right-of-way on the east side of No. 601. From the base, Twin Peaks is clearly in view. From the 50th step the two towers of Golden Gate Bridge coalesce into one.

◢ At the top of Cascade, the street signs read PACHECO 900 FUNSTON 1800. Follow Funston to the right, walking on the odd-numbered side for ocean views between the houses. Next to No. 1850 is a redwood house atop the hill; plantings adorn the wood stairway in front. The cascading garden of succulents is a source of delight for all who stop and look at it. Houses on the odd-numbered side date from the 1970s.

◢ At Aerial (opposite stairway) turn left to Pacheco. Turn right on Pacheco to the triangular piece of land at 12th Ave. and Pacheco. The residents interested in gardening and keeping the neighborhood beautiful have been diligently working together on this project. Ascend the curved stairway to 12th Ave.

◢ Continue left on 12th Ave. to the intersection of Rockridge and Cragmont across from Golden Gate Heights Park. Cross Cragmont and turn left to 12th Ave. At No. 2026 12th Ave. cross the street and follow the paved path into the park. Turn left at the playground and continue right on the path to the roundabout and sitting area at the top. Follow the paved path to descend the hill. Turn left at the tennis courts and continue to Rockridge. Cross Rockridge to Funston.

◢ Carl E. Larsen, a Danish restaurateur, loved this area. His chicken ranch on 17th Ave. and Noriega was the site for the annual Easter Egg Hunt for neighborhood children. By the time of his death in 1924 at age 84, he had given the City six acres of land in Golden Gate Heights, including Golden Gate Heights Park.

◢ Walk on Funston to Aerial Stairway, one of the longest in San Francisco. It is surrounded by cypress trees and ice plant. Descend Aerial Stairway to 14th Ave. at No. 1920. Turn right and continue on 14th Ave.

◢ Now in the 1800 block of 14th Ave., you walk past Ortega Way Stairway next to No. 1883. This is the other side of the hill facing Ortega. Just past the mature acacia, a profile view of the chert outcropping on the Ortega and 14th Ave. hill comes into view. No. 1843 faces directly onto the Franciscan rock outcrop. The rock always reminds me of Nathaniel Hawthorne's short story, "The Great Stone Face." In it, a child, Ernest, spends many hours looking at a rock formation in New Hampshire's White Mountains with his mother. His favorite of her stories was the legend of "a child who should be born hereabouts who was destined to become the greatest and noblest personage of his time, and whose countenance in manhood should bear an exact resemblance to the Great Stone Face." Ernest is recognized as the likeness of the Great Stone Face. As I reflect on this story, two hawks are circling above me.

◢ Next to No. 1795 14th Ave. you descend Mount Stairway, where you may notice that a neighbor has been gardening with native plants. The stairway ends across from No. 1801 15th Ave.

◢ Turn right. Continue on 15th Ave. past Noriega to the retaining wall. Ascend the stairway to upper 15th Ave.

◢ Cross upper 15th Ave. to the Grand View Stairway. Concrete piers support a wood stairway accented by a wood handrail, and a very nicely sited wood-slat bench on the landing allows you to look out west over the ocean. An information placard about Grand View Park is strategically placed at the bottom of the stairs.

◢ Ascend the stairway into Grand View Park, a superb place to watch the sunset. The 1.1-acre park is habitat for several native

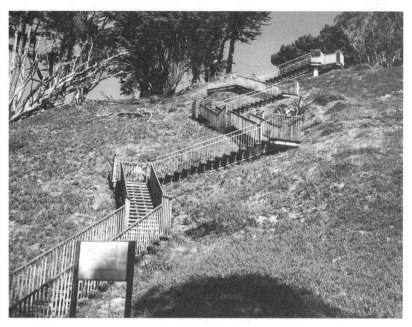

Grand View Park *Peter Nagy*

plant species: bush lupine, beach strawberry, bush monkeyflower, and coyote bush. The rare and endangered plants here are the Franciscan wallflower and the dune tansy. Restoration of Grand View Park is under the aegis of the Yerba Buena chapter of the Native Plant Society and the Natural Areas Division of the City Recreation and Park Department. Both local neighbors and Eagle Scouts participate in volunteer work.

⊿ You will pass two landings with wood benches. At the second bench, take the first footpath to the left for a view of the City. Pass the mature Monterey cypress trees. Continue walking around to the right (the path narrows). Stop and look at the Golden Gate Bridge to observe an optical illusion. I saw what looked like three towers on the Bridge, which changed as I walked around the footpath. As you walk farther, in the distance, Golden Gate Park is a sea of green cutting a swath between the Sunset and Richmond neighborhoods.

⊿ The Veterans Hospital stands on the hill at the farthest point west; and George Washington High School, the large building, is to its east. The curving street that snakes through the park is 19th Ave. St. Anne's Church, with its two spires, is the Sunset neighborhood's most familiar icon. Views to the west feature the Sunset Reservoir and demonstrate the relative flatness of the neighborhood stretching oceanward.

⬛ You're walking on a hill of windblown sand, but underneath it is chert, layered at odd angles, reddish in color, and embedded with pieces of radiolarian, the one-cell marine rhizopod. Geologists have found radiolarian hundreds of feet below sea level and have dated samples at 140 million years. Walking near remnants exposed as the ocean receded, you feel connected to the beginnings of time.

⬛ Continue on the footpath to the stairway. Then turn to look and see that a tower has almost disappeared on the Golden Gate Bridge. Turn left to descend the wood stairway to 14th Ave. At the last landing, a panoramic view from Mt. Sutro to the Golden Gate Bridge. At the bottom of the stairway, now only one tower is visible on the bridge.

⬛ Turn left on 14th Ave. Walk to the intersection of 14th Ave., 15th Ave., and Aloha. Veer left on Aloha to Lomita. At the intersection of Lomita and Aloha, there's a triangular section with a small stairway enhanced by shrubs and flowers. Bear left and descend the stairway to Lomita and continue to 16th Ave. Veer left to your beginning.

Further Ambling

If you wish to go to Golden Gate Park, take MUNI Bus #66 Quintara to 9th Ave. and Judah (two blocks from the park). Points of interest in the park include the San Francisco Botanical Gardens, Conservatory of Flowers, de Young Museum, and the Japanese Tea Garden. Irving is the main shopping street of the Inner Sunset.

Links

St. Francis Wood

& Conundrums

Andrew S. Hallidie's cable car conquered the
Clay St. Hill in 1878 and made Nob Hill accessible.
The Twin Peaks Streetcar Tunnel conquered the West
of Twin Peaks district in 1918 and made the hilly, western area accessible. And that's the beginning of St. Francis
Wood. If you look on a topographic map of the area west of
the Twin Peaks district of San Francisco, you can see why it was
so difficult to develop this side of the range—hills of chert (part of
the Franciscan Formation) and high sand dunes. By implication, it is
an area of wind and fog. But there are the views, the fresh ocean air,
and the forest of trees Adolph Sutro planted after he bought 650 acres
of the Rancho San Miguel land grant in 1880. Sutro was one of the
very few historically important entrepreneurs (Carl Larsen was another) who loved the western part of San Francisco and lived there. Others favored Nob Hill.

Another person who loved the west side of San Francisco was
Duncan McDuffie. He was an environmentalist, president of the Sierra
Club (1928–1931 and 1943–1946), and believed in the principles of the
City Beautiful movement that was gaining momentum throughout
the country in the early 1900s. He also was a partner in the Mason &
McDuffie real estate company. McDuffie enjoyed the western section
of San Francisco, and the company was interested in purchasing land
here. The only amenity missing was good transportation.

Michael O'Shaughnessy, chief engineer at the time, proposed building the Twin Peaks Streetcar Tunnel to solve this City problem. Finally,

in 1912, construction began. Real estate developers began to buy land. Mason & McDuffie bought 175 acres of the Rancho San Miguel from the four Sutro heirs who were free to sell after their father's will was declared null and void. Mason & McDuffie planned to develop St. Francis Wood.

The company had previously developed several neighborhoods in Berkeley, Crescent Park, Claremont Upland, and Park Hills that expressed the idea of open space, trees, shrubs, and parks as important ingredients in designing a city neighborhood that is pleasing and nourishing for the human being. Mason & McDuffie planned St. Francis Wood in the same spirit with circular streets, spaces between houses, wide sidewalks, parks, open space, and lots of trees. The company hired the finest landscape designers, the Frederick Law Olmsted, Jr. office of Boston, and the architects were associated with the Department of Architecture at the University of California, Berkeley. During World War I, business was marginal. (In 1915, the company's total income amounted to $5,000.) McDuffie persisted in his vision of nature and city living. Loans from friendly banks helped. After the first streetcar ran through the tunnel in 1918, business increased. By 1925, more than 400 families were living in St. Francis Wood.

The circular streets and open spaces are not exactly circular (I use *circular* loosely because mathematicians only allow 360° to a circle.) St. Francis Wood has, in some places, an irrational street design, as an architect friend described it. A street can diverge into two directions, but the two segments share the same name. To find your way without losing the rhythm of the walk, be sure to look for the numbers on the street signs, such as SAN PABLO 300 or SANTA PAULA 70.

◢ There are several entrances into St. Francis Wood. You will enter through one of the back doors so that you will end close to the beginning of the walk. There are two alternatives. You can begin on the north side of Portola Drive at the border of the Edgehill neighborhood on Ulloa and Kensington, where there are no parking restrictions except for street cleaning. Walk across the Portola pedestrian overpass to Miraloma and Marne on the south side of Portola. This is my favorite and most unusual beginning of the walk. The second alternative is to come by bus and begin at the pedestrian overpass at Miraloma near Marne.

◢ If you elect the first alternative, you will see an aged Monterey pine, with multiple trunks and cascading branches, that provides a canopy for the overpass. The West of Twin Peaks district is a forest of sub-neighborhoods—West Portal, Monterey Heights, Mt. Davidson, Sherwood Forest, and others. In spite of this and the hilly terrain, lot sizes are spacious, and the sensation of space is augmented by vegetation. Look across Ulloa toward the Edgehill neighborhood, a beautiful scene.

◢ Make a right turn on Miraloma toward No. 2 Miraloma. It is a very large house with a tiled roof and fits in comfortably with the corner. Look around and you will see the tip of the cross on Mt. Davidson. Descend the short stairway on the right to Portola. The traffic noise level on Portola is a reminder to listen and compare noise levels as you walk throughout the City. At the bottom of the stairway, you come to an unusual sight. The New Zealand Christmas tree, *Metrosideros excelsus*, at the base of the stairway

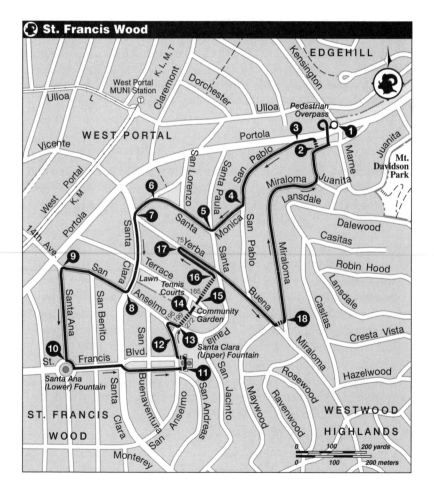

WALK 12 ROUTE: St. Francis Wood

Public Transportation: MUNI Bus #43 Masonic and #48 Quintara. Farther away, several Metro lines stop at West Portal Station. For Muni bus or Metro information, call 311 (outside San Francisco call (415) 701-2311).

Parking: You can park on Ulloa at Kensington with no restrictions of time, except on the day for garbage pickup.

1. At Portola, take pedestrian overpass from Kensington to Miraloma. Right on Miraloma.
2. Before No. 2 Miraloma, descend stairway to Portola and left to San Pablo.
3. Left on San Pablo to Santa Monica.
4. Cross street and walk right onto Santa Monica to Santa Paula.
5. Continue right on Santa Monica. (Check the street signs carefully.)
6. Pass San Lorenzo and follow curve to the left on Santa Monica to Santa Clara.
7. Left on Santa Clara to San Anselmo.
8. Right on San Anselmo to Santa Ana.
9. Sharp left on Santa Ana to St. Francis Blvd. and the Santa Ana Fountain (or Lower Fountain) and roundabout.
10. Left on St. Francis Blvd. Pass San Benito and San Buenaventura to San Anselmo and the St. Francis Blvd. Fountain (or Upper Fountain) and plaza.
11. Ascend the stairway to the right. Walk toward the left. Descend stairway on your left. Right to street sign that reads SAN ANSELMO 200 and SANTA PAULA END.
12. Walk on San Anselmo past the white fire hydrant No. 6 and trees. Cross San Anselmo to No. 195 and continue right to No. 199.
13. Immediately after No. 199, turn left to descend Terrace Walk Stwy.
14. Right to walk around the community herbal garden to 165 Terrace Drive.
15. Ascend the continuation of Terrace Walk Stwy. At the end of Terrace Walk you will be directly across from street sign 100 YERBA BUENA.
16. Left on Yerba Buena to Nos. 75, 44, and 34.
17. Retrace your steps to the 100 YERBA BUENA street sign and continue past Santa Paula and San Pablo. Just past Maywood, ascend stairway on the left to Miraloma.
18. Left on Miraloma to your beginning.

Linking

If you wish to link St. Francis Wood with Mt. Davidson (Walk 13), walk to Marne and Miraloma. Proceed with directions for Walk 13.

Another graceful link can be made with Edgehill (Walk 14). Walk across the pedestrian overpass at Portola and Miraloma to Kensington. Turn right on Ulloa and proceed with directions for Walk 14.

has red aerial roots that travel down the trunk of the host tree until they touch ground. At that time, they start to develop into a separate trunk, much like a banyan tree. This only occurs in areas where there is optimum fog and dampness. Another area in the City where you will find an example of this is at the entrance of the San Francisco Botanical Garden, opposite the Japanese Tea Garden and adjacent to Stow Lake.

◢ As you walk left on Portola you will see a sign POSITIVELY NO TRESPASSING at the bottom of a discontinued, derelict stairway. Next to it is No. 1135, beautifully terraced with rocks. A standard with a light on top is next to the garage. The street sign here reads PORTOLA 1200 SAN PABLO 000. Walk to San Pablo following the curve. Pass another entrance that has a concrete standard inscribed with the name ST. FRANCIS WOOD. On the hilly part of the left sidewalk on which you are walking, there are unusual mounds of English ivy. The eucalyptus ficifolia is the street tree here. They are abloom with orange blossoms usually in August and September. There is variety in the house roofs from deeply sloped to roofs that extend to the hip of the house. The sidewalk has little insets of brick squares. There is abundant foliage, an inviting entrance to the neighborhood.

Traveler, there is no path. Paths are made by walking.
—Antonio Machado y Ruiz

◢ You cross the street onto Santa Monica where the street sign reads SANTA MONICA END. Continue to Santa Paula. At the intersection, at No. 101 Santa Monica, is a house of many gables. I tested myself to see if I counted the same number three times in a row. How many do you count?

◢ Continue to the right on Santa Monica where the house numbers are below 100. The direction of the curving streets is confusing, so check the signs carefully. Pass No. 94 on the left, and take a look at No. 90 (the number is on the side of the house). This English style house, built of natural concrete in 1921, has a low wavy wood roof and mullion windows. It was designed by Henry Gutterson. The present occupants are only the second owners of the home. When they moved in, they had the roof reshingled. They asked the roofers to save the moss which they then donated to the collection of the Strybing Arboretum, now officially known as the San Francisco Botanical Garden at Strybing Arboretum.

- Across the street, No. 85 Santa Monica is another Gutterson English style stone house, built from Idaho sandstone in 1925. It is one of my favorite houses in St. Francis Wood. The house is angled and next to it is a large hydrangea plant. A St. Francis sculpture is niched near the front door. The landscaping around the house is tastefully constructed with a variety of shapes of foliage and a variety of trees, the oldest of which dates back to the 1890s, when Sutro planted them.

- At the intersection of San Lorenzo on the left, the street sign states SANTA MONICA 50. In the center of the street, there is an open space with benches. New trees have been planted, and some old, enormous Monterey pines are established here. At the V-shaped part of this rounded triangle, there are two street signs—SANTA MONICA 33–55 and SANTA MONICA 30. Walk on Santa Monica 30. A short, but useful stairway was built at No. 30 Santa Monica with six slabs of concrete that lead into the backyard.

- At the corner of Santa Monica and Santa Clara No. 40, turn left. Cross the street at the sign that reads YERBA BUENA 000, and walk on the right side of Santa Clara past Terrace. The St. Francis Wood Home Association office blends imperceptibly into its environment at No. 101 Santa Clara. A park and playground surround the structure in the back. All homeowners are members of the association that manages community property—parks, gardens, tennis courts, gateways, and The Children's Common in the public areas.

- Continue walking on Santa Clara to San Anselmo. Turn right on San Anselmo to walk to Santa Ana. London Plane trees line the length of San Anselmo. Originally the developers wanted to have each circle block have the same street trees and the same style houses, but the plan was not entirely successful. At Santa Ana, make a sharp left. The trees along the street here are ficus. Hebe was planted near the curve. Santa Ana is one of the flat streets and was one of the first developments in St. Francis Wood. The canopy of vegetation is sparse because many of the trees have only recently been planted. Compared to other streets, it seems almost bare.

- You are now at Santa Ana No. 100 and St. Francis Blvd. No. 300, the location of the Santa Ana Fountain (the residents call it the Lower Fountain) and roundabout. It was designed by supervising architect John Galen Howard, dean of the School of Architecture at the University of California, Berkeley from 1903 to 1924. He also designed the pillar entrances and sidewalk patterns. Short stairways are at every corner of the roundabout. Turn left at the fountain onto St. Francis Blvd. The light standard reads THE CIRCLE. Continue left on St. Francis Blvd., and walk past the corner of San Benito No. 100 and St. Francis Blvd. No. 400.

◢ Continue on St. Francis Blvd. The traffic on the boulevard is heavy. There are stop signs on some of the corners, but watch and be aware. Use the crosswalks. When I began exploring the St. Francis Wood neighborhood, I was impressed by the number, the sizes, the ages, and the variety of trees, especially the eucalyptus, on St. Francis Blvd. From a distance the lines of trees seem to continue forever, and in a sense, they will. Some of the trees were brought in from the 1915 Panama Pacific International Exposition.

◢ The houses on the boulevard are formal and stately. No. 405 St. Francis Blvd. dates to 1948. You are now at St. Francis Blvd. No. 500 and Santa Clara No. 300. Cross Santa Clara and continue on St. Francis Blvd. A large oval median is the introduction to the ornamented St. Francis Blvd. Fountain (or Upper Fountain as the residents call it) designed by Gutterson in 1912. A mature magnolia flourishes at No. 531. You can see the Brush cherry trees near the corner of San Buenaventura where they line the street near No. 50. No. 600 St. Francis Blvd. is a stucco house, with curved living room windows extending almost down to grass level. Baroque decoration surrounds the front door. No. 630 St. Francis Blvd. is built in the southwest architectural style with overhangs against the sun.

◢ You arrive at the St. Francis Blvd. Fountain (Upper Fountain as the residents call it) at San Anselmo. There are stone benches on each side of the boulevard for you to take your time to enjoy the long view of the fountain within its setting. St. Francis Blvd. is the main axis and the imposing main entrance of the neighborhood with streets radiating from it. Walk across San Anselmo to the plaza area. All around the walkway by the plaza are red brick squares inscribed with the names of donors who contributed to the 1998 restoration of the plaza's sculptured features, like the fountain. On the left side of the wall is a plaque with a portrait of Duncan McDuffie and a tribute to his vision for St. Francis Wood.

◢ Ascend the stairway on your right near San Andreas. Walk left past the fountain and plaza area and descend the stairway to the left. Turn right to the intersection where the street sign reads SANTA PAULA END and SAN ANSELMO 200. Continue walking on San Anselmo, past the white fire hydrant No. 6, and the stand of 12 London Plane trees. This is where the fun begins!

- Cross San Anselmo and turn right to No. 195. Walk past No. 199 and immediately turn left to the entrance of Terrace Walk Stairway, which begins with a gravel-lined pathway with shrubbery all around. (Incidentally, if you walk beyond No. 199 San Anselmo, you are then on Santa Paula.)

- The stairway is well situated here in terms of the rhythm and length of the walk. Descend this stairway of redwood steps, which feels more pliant to the feet than other types of wood. The landings are concrete and the railings are metal. Assorted foliage is growing around the sides. The stairway descends to No. 266 Terrace Drive. A community herbal garden is on the right, a tool shed is in the center, and tennis courts are on the left.

- The Terrace Walk Stairway continues on the left side of No. 165 Terrace Drive. Ascend the stairway onto a pathway to the street. You will be directly across from a street sign YERBA BUENA 100. Turn left to No. 75 Yerba Buena, a house designed by Julia Morgan and built on a rise. A curved brick stairway leads up to the front door framed with Corinthian columns. The house has a more formal appearance than other houses on the block. The windows are wall length.

- Walk to No. 44 to see the delicate filagree gate. A eucalyptus tree with an impressive and unusual gall-like swelling is in front of No. 34. The growth appears to have been caused by a cellular division that went out of control—somewhat analogous to cancer but not as serious. The leaves from the eucalyptus trees on this block were formerly picked by the San Francisco Zoo to feed the koala bears. At the present time, the horticulture staff collects branches every day from various areas of the City, including McLaren Park, Visitacion Valley, Stern Grove, Candlestick Park, and Monterey Blvd. The koalas are finicky eaters and are offered at least five different varieties of eucalyptus every day.

- Return to Santa Paula and continue walking on Yerba Buena. Pass San Pablo on your left, and continue on Yerba Buena toward Miraloma. No. 136 Yerba Buena has a very attractive stone chimney. Looking at it instantly reminds me of childhood summer camp, sitting around a cheery fireplace, making smores. Continue on Yerba Buena past Maywood. Ascend the stairway on the left at the MIRALOMA END sign. Continue walking left on Miraloma to your beginning.

Now You See It,

Mt. Davidson

Now You Don't:
Discover the Fog & Light
of San Francisco

Mt. Davidson is part of the enormous area west
of Twin Peaks, and is surrounded by sub-neigh-
borhood sections: Sherwood Forest (there's a Robin
Hood Drive here), Westwood Highlands, and Miraloma
Park. Larger homes can be found west and north of Mt.
Davidson, the smaller ones in the eastern Miraloma section.
Feel free to ramble through the various surrounding neighbor-
hoods. You will see magnificent views beside Miraloma School at
Omar and Myra, and from Marietta Drive and Bella Vista.

At 938', Mt. Davidson is the highest hill in San Francisco. Known
in the 1850s as Blue Mountain, it was renamed Mt. Davidson in 1911
to honor George Davidson (1825–1911), first surveyor of the mountain,
internationally renowned scientist, and president of the California
Academy of Sciences. Mt. Davidson became a city park in December
1929.

The idea of a cross on Mt. Davidson originated with James Decatur,
and an Easter service was first held there in 1923. At that time there

was a 40-foot wood cross, which was replaced three times over the years. Finally, in 1934, the present 100-foot stone cross was erected with a time capsule and the original deed to Mt. Davidson placed in the base. One week before Easter of that year, President Franklin Roosevelt lit the cross via telegraph. The City annually illuminated it during Christmas and Easter seasons, and thousands of people have attended the Easter Sunday sunrise services. In 1996, the U.S. Appeals Court ruled that the religious symbol violates the constitutional separation of church and state. In 1997, San Francisco approved the sale of the cross and surrounding one-third acre to the Armenian American Organization of Northern California for $26,000. It is to be preserved as a historic landmark in memory of the 1.5 million Armenian victims of genocide perpetrated by the Turkish government from 1915 to 1918.

Walking the trails that cut across slopes covered with pine and eucalyptus can be confusing because the Department of Recreation and Parks has not yet put up signage. My challenge was finding the trail leading to the desired exit. Though I tried the walk at different times with various friends, the problem continued. An engineer friend finally solved it by advising, "Keep it simple." It worked. We found two beautiful stone stairways, the breathtaking view, trails with blackberries (edible) and Coast strawberries (inedible), ferns, and wildflowers—forget-me-nots, nasturtiums, and monkeyflowers. Breathing ocean air and eucalyptus, we were in the City but also quite removed from it.

While historic trail names are extant from 1935, when the Works Progress Administration trail-blazed Mt. Davidson, without signage I've resorted to two nonhistoric names. Sherwood Trail is named for the street at the end of the trail. The Native Garden Trail was always a footpath and not included in the original park.

◢ Begin west of Mt. Davidson, at the stone stairway next to No. 275 Juanita. Your route is upward. Blackberries growing along the stairway are delicious in season. When you reach a nonfunctioning drinking fountain (still useful as a landmark), ascend toward the right. At the next fork, climb toward the left. Wildflowers grow alongside the trail. Where the Cresta Vista Trail joins your route on the left, near the tall sequoia tree, ascend to the right. Where the Native Garden Trail joins your trail at the point of a switchback, turn sharply right to continue up the Juanita Trail to Saint Croix Road.

Cross Saint Croix Road (for vehicles). Ascend the stone stairway, turn left and continue on the log stairway. Turn right, and ascend the tree root and log stairway behind the cross to the summit. At the summit, walk to the front of the cross toward the cliff side, where you will see views of the East Bay hills and the Campanile (Sather Tower) at UC Berkeley.

Turn left and descend the wood stairway. Follow the East Ridge Trail to the panoramic viewpoint. Retrace your steps, but bear left before the wood stairway. Descend and continue along a medium-steep gravel and log path, the Sherwood Trail.

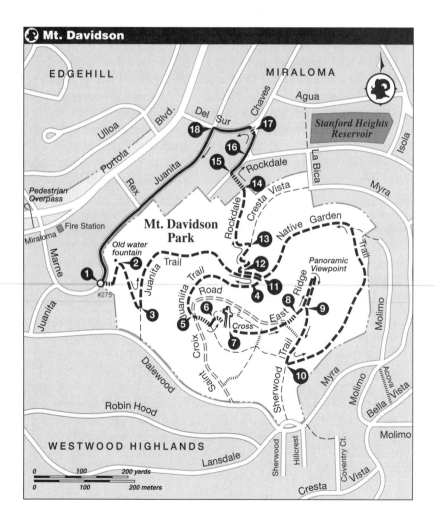

WALK 13 ROUTE: Mt. Davidson

Public Transportation: MUNI Bus #43 Masonic and #48 Quintara. Farther away several Metro lines stop at West Portal Station. For MUNI bus or Metro information, call 311 (outside San Francisco call (415) 701-2311).

Note: Portions of the trails are narrow and rocky. Watch your step. The park is under reconstruction. Information here is the latest available.

1. Follow Marne from Miraloma to your beginning at No. 275 Juanita. Ascend the stone stairway beside the house.

2. Left on Juanita Trail. Right at the nonfunctioning drinking fountain.

3. Turn left and ascend the trail. Where Cresta Vista Trail joins your route on the left by the tall sequoia tree, continue up toward the right.

4. At junction (ahead) with Native Garden Trail, switchback right, staying on the Juanita Trail.

5. Cross the access (Saint Croix) road, and ascend a stone stairway and then log stairway bearing left.

6. Right and ascend a log stairway to the back of the cross on the summit.

7. Walk to front of the cross toward cliff side.

8. Left and descend wood stairway. Follow the East Ridge Trail to the panoramic overlook.

9. Retrace your steps to the first left. Descend south on a medium-steep gravel and log road, the Sherwood Trail.

10. After the fifth log, bear left on the Native Garden Trail, which descends and partly circumnavigates the peak. Ascend a tree root stairway.

11. Where the Native Garden Trail joins the Juanita Trail at the switchback, turn right to descend.

12. Right at the first path, Cresta Vista Trail, across from the tall sequoia tree. It switchbacks a couple times before reaching the junction with the Rockdale Trail.

13. Left at junction onto Rockdale Trail. Path narrows just before the stairway.

14. Descend stone stairway to Rockdale St.

15. Right on Rockdale St.

16. Left on Chaves. Descend corner stairway to Del Sur.

17. Left on Del Sur to Juanita.

18. Left on Juanita to your beginning.

Linking

If you wish to link Mt. Davidson with Edgehill (Walk 14), walk across the overhead pedestrian skyway at Portola and Miraloma to Kensington. Turn right on Ulloa and proceed with directions for Walk 14.

Another graceful link can be made with St. Francis Wood (Walk 12) by walking to Marne and Miraloma. Proceed with directions for Walk 12.

◢ Soon after the fifth log where the Sherwood Trail meets the Native Garden Trail, turn left. The trail descends and partly circumnavigates the peak, overlooking the Miraloma Park neighborhood. You will pass two high wire fences and ascend a tree root stairway. Watch your step. The barren path leads to the wooded area that eventually rejoins the Juanita Trail.

◢ At the junction, turn right to descend Juanita Trail. Almost immediately you reach the junction of Cresta Vista Trail. Look for the tall sequoia tree. Turn right down the Cresta Vista Trail. It gently veers left and right a couple times before reaching the junction with the Rockdale Trail.

Jamaicans don't say, "Goodbye." They say, "Walk good."

◢ Turn left onto Rockdale Trail. Cross over a log buried in the path. It has a yellow reflector attached to it. Continue on the path to a stone stairway that ends on Rockdale St. Turn right on Rockdale. Veer left on Chaves and descend corner stairway to Del Sur. Turn left to Juanita to your beginning. On the way you pass Franciscan Formation outcrops at the park's edge, and some seeps (active in winter) that encourage ferns, eucalyptus, and other lush vegetation.

Further Ambling

Two other entrances to the park are the Saint Croix Trail at No. 39 Dalewood, and the Sherwood Trail at the #36 Teresita MUNI bus stop on Dalewood. The Saint Croix Trail has two stone stairways ascending to the summit. (Another stone stairway is closed at this time.) An upper stone stairway is near Juanita Trail. Beyond this stairway on Saint Croix Trail to the summit is a large rock outcropping with hanging greenery. The Sherwood Trail meets East Ridge Trail and the Native Garden Trail.

To traverse Mt. Davidson and exit by another trailhead, from the summit follow the East Ridge Trail to the panoramic lookout and partly retrace your steps to descend along the first left-branching road, the Sherwood Trail. Keep going ahead where the Native Garden Trail branches left. You can descend the Sherwood Trail down to Myra and Dalewood, where you can take MUNI Bus #36 Teresita to Forest Hill Station or the Balboa Park BART station.

You could also walk left on Myra around the park on the city streets to La Bica. Turn right on La Bica, walk one block to Rockdale, turn left for a block, and then continue, as described above, to your beginning at No. 275 Juanita.

Chert, Hideaway Paths,

Edgehill

& Open Space

The Edgehill houses perched 600 feet above sea
level allow their occupants extraordinary sunsets,
glistening Pacific Ocean waters, and 32 miles to the
northwest, sightings of the Farallon Islands, which are
part of the sovereignty of San Francisco. In return for these
favors of nature, the residents have accepted narrow roads
and troublesome curves, as well as periodic landslides. The fire
department has learned to send up extra lengths of hose, and not to
send up the hook and ladder truck. Delivery companies likewise do
not send up large trucks. Developers have learned to expect noisy
opposition from residents to their plans for building more homes on
precarious portions of land. Still, a few developments have been built
on the precipices. And problems have arisen.

The most recent major one occurred in 1997 when residents noticed
cracks in the road that increased in size the next day. Under the direction of consulting engineers and geologists, Cotton, Shires, & Associates, Inc., crews worked vigorously to stabilize Edgehill Way and
prevent more damage to homes at both the top edge and the bottom of
the cliff. Several residents were forced to vacate their homes. The story
will unfold as you walk, beginning at the base of the circle, from bottom to top, from the newest addition to the oldest.

◢ Begin at Ulloa and Waithman, the entrance to Knockash Hill Rd.,
and walk through the pedestrian gate. This development of 13

homes, also known as the Knockash neighborhood, has undergone a metamorphosis since I began to explore the area in the 1980s. It was a parking lot, and the church was the only structure here. (I included a description of it in the third edition.) But before that, it was the site of a stone quarry. After the horrific rockslide in January 1997, I felt I should wait until geologic conditions became more stable before I included another Edgehill walk. In 2005, I came back to scout the area—alone, with friends, and with people interested in seeing the neighborhood. Knockash Hill Rd. was a dramatic surprise. I felt I wanted to include an Edgehill walk and that I had no choice but to begin the walk at Ulloa and Waithman.

◢ My first reaction was: "How beautiful!" On my right, within 20 feet of where I stand, is a wall of layered red chert—of chert built up over the last 100 million years. My second reaction was: "Where did all these houses come from?" What a contrast in age between the 100-million-year-old wall and this new human-made walkway and brick border on my left—within 20 feet of each other.

◢ I enjoyed my research—talking with residents and reading in the main branch of the City library. The quarry work in the early 20th century had intensified the fragility of the steep cliffs, resulting in small rock falls. The cliffs were not successfully stabilized until after the 1997 landslide. You see the wire mesh that covers the slope as you walk through Knockash. It's difficult for me to visualize how it was done, but according to the records, 99 multistrand, double-corrosion-protected tieback anchors were used, and almost 1,200 linear feet of belt structures are part of the stabilization plan.

◢ The grey specks in the chert are radiolarian, an aquatic plankton. Chert, one of the elements of the Franciscan Formation, was pushed up from deep water by volcanic upheavals. (You can see good examples of it around the parking lot of the Randall Museum, south of Corona Heights.) Succulents grow on the hillside, and lichens abound on the rocks. A bit farther on, you see the formation on both sides of the street.

◢ Pillars on the left and right sides of the road introduce the New Life Church of the Nazarene. The congregation here is relatively small (church headquarters are in Kansas City, Missouri), but the group observes the main tenet—holiness. This is achieved by ministering to the homeless, and helping them to lead, eventually, a life of holiness by serving others less fortunate. The church celebrated its 100th anniversary in 2005. The hillside is terraced, and a small area is allocated for church parking.

- At the cul-de-sac end of Knockash Hill Rd. are two basketball hoops. (Young couples with children comprise the majority of homeowners in the Knockash subdivision.) Continue up toward the right on a narrowing path. There are two pillars and a sign that reads EDGEHILL MOUNTAIN OPEN SPACE, SAN FRANCISCO RECREATION AND PARKS.

- Knockash Hill Rd. is one of the entrances into the park. A descending dirt path introduces you to a wooded area. The path leads to corner pie-shaped steps behind a sitting area. Bear right on the upper path to walk on the rustic stairway that wends among the trees and leads to the residential area.

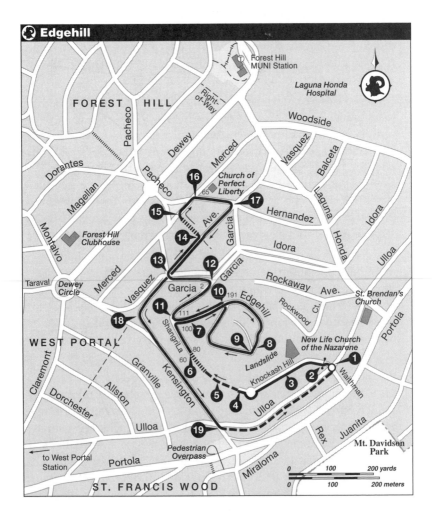

WALK 14 ROUTE: Edgehill

Public Transportation: MUNI Bus #43 Masonic and #48 Quintara. Farther away, several Metro lines stop at Forest Hill Station. For MUNI bus or Metro information, call 311 (outside San Francisco call (415) 701-2311).

Parking: Unlimited parking is available on Ulloa at Kensington.

Note: The Farallon Islands can be seen on a clear day from Ulloa and Kensington. It's spectacular at sunset.

1. Begin at Ulloa and Waithman.
2. Enter resident gate of Knockash neighborhood. Walk on left side of street.
3. Walk past New Life Church of the Nazarene on the right and Knockash Hill residences on the left.
4. Bear right at Edgehill Mountain Open Space Area sign onto path.
5. From the top proceed downhill a few feet, and follow the upper path/ stairway to your right.
6. The Open Space area ends at No. 60 on ShangriLa Way (unmarked). Continue to the end of Shangrila Way to No. 100 Edgehill Way and turn right.
7. Continue up Edgehill Way, and follow the one-way sign around the mountain.
8. Pass No. 280 and continue past the mailboxes, Nos. 300 and 350 Edgehill, and the driveway to the right, which is private property and closed to public walking.
9. Continue past fire hydrant labeled No. 8 and walk through wooded area.
10. Left at No. 191 Edgehill Way and backtrack to No. 111 Edgehill Way.
11. Right at No. 111 Edgehill Way to No. 2 Upper Garcia.
12. Left on Upper Garcia to Vasquez.
13. Right on Vasquez to Pacheco.
14. Left on Pacheco and descend stairway to Merced.
15. Right on Merced to Hernandez.
16. Right on Hernandez to Vasquez.
17. Right on Vasquez to Kensington.
18. Sharp left on Kensington to Ulloa.
19. Left on Ulloa to your beginning.

Linking

If you wish to link Edgehill with Forest Hill (Walk 15), after Step 14 above, cross Merced to Dewey Blvd. and then follow directions for Walk 15. On your return, cross Dewey Blvd. to Merced, and continue Walk 14 with Step 15, to your beginning.

Another graceful link can be made with Mt. Davidson (Walk 13) by walking across the pedestrian overpass at Portola and Kensington to Miraloma and then following the directions for Walk 13.

◢ A bench, a bit off the path, is an invitation to those who would like to sit and contemplate the serene setting of blue gum eucalyptus and Monterey pine and cypress and the height and steepness of the slopes. Every month, dedicated volunteers plant native plants and grass, a successful venture; they also rid the area of invasive plants like ehrharta grass and ivy. Blue, yellow, and white flags mark sites of new plantings. Walk up log steps where wild onions sprout on the side of the stairs.

◢ As you come to the edge of the open space, you are on ShangriLa Way. Its existence invites a great trivia question: What is the shortest 'street' in the City that, although without signage has a legal name known to the residents but not to outsiders. The answer is ShangriLa Way. It extends from house No. 60 to the metal horse at house No. 100, a distance of only a few feet. The rest of Edgehill has one name—Edgehill Way. ShangriLa is the second entrance into the Open Space Park.

◢ No. 60 ShangriLa Way at the top of the hill, on your left, is built on steel stilts. No. 80 (on the right side) has an unusually long window wall. The owners of No. 56 enjoy a compelling view to the north, complemented by a patio. A bit farther on is No. 54 with an unusual exterior of concrete embedded with pebbles.

◢ No. 100 Edgehill and ShangriLa is unusual because of the two sculptures at the corner. You first pass a totem pole fabricated by a member of a Native American tribe in Washington State; the metal bear comes from Mexico. You are now on Edgehill Way.

◢ As you turn right, you come across No. 111, one of the largest homes on the hill. No. 140 on the right side has beautiful stone steps from the quarry. Across the street, on the other side of No. 121, you can see the canyon below. It is wild with trees and vines, nasturtium, wild onion, and some California poppies. No. 191 is at the end where the road around the mountain begins. No. 200 has a stone wall that I find particularly appealing. No. 220, in the early days, was a speakeasy. No. 250 was the first house built on the hill in 1927 by the current resident's father. It incorporates, so pleasingly, huge boulders on the property (even embedding a mailbox into one) and redwood trees. The stones that are an integral part of the architecture of many homes here come from the quarry.

◢ On my walks through the neighborhood, I met neighbors out for their daily walks. Soon, I noticed that we were walking in a group.

Several of them have lived in Edgehill for close to 50 years. They love living on the mountain.

Edgehill neighborhood was one of my husband's favorite areas in San Francisco. We lived there for 46 years. We saw the Farallon Islands on a clear day. We could see Golden Gate Bridge, the two tunnels beyond, and Forest Hills with its colorful houses and tile roofs that reminded us of the hill towns of Italy. We did have a lot of fog, but even then, it was very beautiful. The sunsets were magnificent. Sometimes they were orange, sometimes pink—there isn't a more beautiful place in San Francisco on a nice day.

—Former resident J. M.

◢ The area between Nos. 275 and 301 is the site of the 1997 mudslide that destroyed part of the street and where a small modern house with solar heating was formerly located. After the slide, it was declared unsafe for occupancy, taken down, and destroyed. The retaining wall and the additional metal fencing was erected as part of the stabilizing plan.

◢ From No. 280 continue past the private driveway with mailboxes Nos. 300 and 350, and the white water hydrant with the number 8 printed on it. Continue walking into the wooded area of Edgehill Way.

◢ This is one of the most magical unblocks in San Francisco—a *rus in urbe* (the country in the city), if one can ever use the term—*Here in Edgehill, I am suddenly transported. I am walking a narrow path, one-car wide, confined by a deep ravine on my left, enclosed by the chert wall on my right, from which trees are hanging randomly, eucalyptus and pine. I feel I am treading lightly on soft easy earth. But I'm not. I am walking on macadam. On the edges of the road, I see the layers of brick on the right side of the road that had been used previously on the property.* San Francisco accepted it from the developer only as a public road to be driven on; it did not accept the responsibility for maintenance—catch-22.

◢ At No. 345 we're back in the City. Turn left at No. 191. At No. 111 Edgehill, veer to your right and continue walking downhill to Garcia. (At Garcia near Edgehill Way in January 1995, 250 Pacific Gas & Electric customers were without power after a 60-foot tree fell on the roof of a nearby building.) Continue left on Garcia to Vasquez.

◢ Turn right at No. 150 to descend the little Pacheco Stairway, a series of steps and landings. The widest steps are at the base of Merced, where benches are built into the wall. As you descend you become conscious of how this stairway echoes the longer Pacheco Stairway in front of you (the Forest Hill neighborhood).

◢ Turn right on Merced until you come to Hernandez. The Church of Perfect Liberty at No. 65 Merced occupies a large white structure at the corner, a former residence. It has been in San Francisco since 1960 and has a congregation of 250 to 300 persons. Perfect Liberty is a religious group founded in Japan in 1924 by Tokuharu Miki, who died in 1938. The church's mission is to bring about world peace by living the precepts of "Life is Art" and "Man's life is a succession of self-expressions."

◢ Continue right on Hernandez, and turn right on Vasquez to Kensington. Turn left to Ulloa and left to your beginning.

Marienbad

Forest Hill

in San Francisco

It's not the longest stairway in the City, or the steepest; not the most charming, or the most personal. Filbert and Vallejo Stairways, Oakhurst Stairway, Vulcan and Harry Stairways, and Pemberton Stairway, respectively, have these attributes.

However, the grand Pacheco Stairway is by far the most elegant in San Francisco. An urn of flowers 20 feet in diameter introduces this long stairway placed amidst forest and lawns. The stairs themselves—18 feet wide, with balustrades, columns, and patterns of stones repeating into the distance—lend a dreamlike, rococo quality to the setting. Think of Alain Resnais's film *Last Year at Marienbad*; and how easily the Pacheco Stairway could fit the surroundings of Marienbad. This walk of curves and curlicues reiterates the innate elegance of this stairway in its Forest Hill setting.

Forest Hill was originally part of the 4,000-acre Rancho San Miguel, granted in 1843 to José de Jesús Noe, the last Mexican *alcalde* (Spanish for *mayor*) of San Francisco. After California became part of the United States, the 11 ranchos that comprised the town were subdivided. In 1880 Adolph Sutro bought 1,100 acres of Noe's rancho; the Crocker Estate bought the rest.

Public transportation became easily accessible to the western part of the City after the Twin Peaks Tunnel was built. In anticipation of this, the Newell-Murdoch Company began subdividing the Forest Hill tract in 1912, cutting down much of what had been extremely dense forest planted by Adolph Sutro and his Arbor Day volunteers. Difficult engineering and construction problems were solved in a most aesthetic manner by Mark Daniels, the landscape engineer (and former General Superintendent of the U.S. National Parks), who deserves a plaque commending his design of curving streets that follow terrain contours, generous stairways, ornamental urns, concrete benches, balustrades, parks, and terraces.

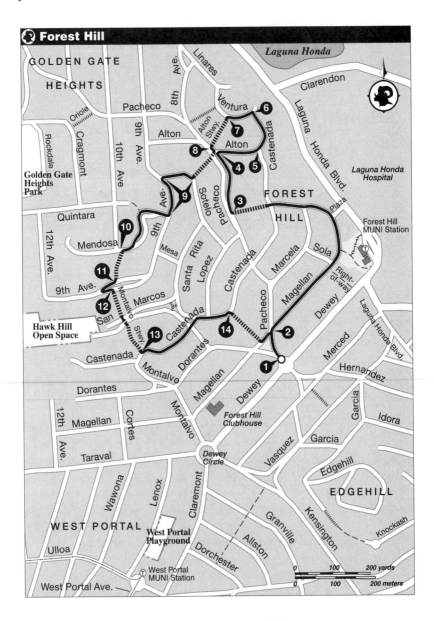

Forest Hill also has the distinction of having the largest concentration of Bernard Maybeck homes in the City. Maybeck is my favorite California architect of the early 1900s who espoused the Craftsman style of architecture. He used redwood for the exteriors, brought light into the interiors, and he related living areas to gardens. Maybeck taught in the School of Architecture at the University of California, Berkeley. He died in 1957 at the age of 95.

No. 266 Pacheco was the first house built in Forest Hill (1913). In 1918, the year the first streetcar went through the Twin Peaks Tunnel, the Forest Hill Association was organized. They set home-building standards such as a minimum 1,500-square-foot interior and 19-foot setback from the sidewalk. They taxed themselves to maintain the grounds; and because the streets and stairways, delightful and

WALK 15 ROUTE: Forest Hill

Public Transportation: MUNI Metro L, M, or K to Forest Hill Station; #43 Masonic; #44 O'Shaughnessy. For MUNI bus or Metro information, call 311 (outside San Francisco call (415) 701-2311).

1. Begin at Dewey and Pacheco. Walk to Magellan.
2. Right on Magellan past Sola and Marcela to the stairway next to No. 140 Castenada. Ascend to No. 334 Pacheco.
3. Right on Pacheco to Alton.
4. Right on Alton to Castenada.
5. Left on Castenada to Ventura.
6. Left on Ventura to No. 60 Ventura.
7. Ascend stairway to Pacheco, No. 400.
8. Cross the street to crosswalk at Pacheco and Alton street sign. Walk up 10 steps to upper Pacheco and cross street to No. 399 Pacheco. Continue ascending Alton Stwy.
9. At the top of stairway, next to No. 60 Sotelo, bear right, then left on 9th Ave., and right on Mendosa.
10. Descend the Montalvo Stwy. between Nos. 91 and 99 Mendosa.
11. Curve right around planted median, then left to lower 9th Ave., next to No. 2238 9th Ave.
12. Descend Montalvo Stwy. on lower 9th Ave. past San Marcos to Castenada.
13. Left on Castenada to grand Pacheco Stwy. next to No. 249 Castenada.
14. Descend to Pacheco and Dewey to your beginning.

Linking

To link Forest Hill with Edgehill (Walk 14), cross Dewey Blvd. to Merced. Turn left and follow Edgehill route Steps 16–19. Then follow Edgehill route Steps 1–14 to return to your beginning at Dewey and Pacheco.

nonconforming, did not meet city specifications, the association was also responsible for them. After years of controversy and court action, the City, in 1978, accepted responsibility for streets and curbs in Forest Hill, but the residents remain responsible for stairways and sidewalks. The association is still an active community group, which meets regularly at the Forest Hill Clubhouse.

▪ Begin the walk at Dewey and Pacheco. Walk north on Pacheco to Magellan; turn right and walk on the right side of Magellan. The trees and the uniform height of the homes provide a counterpoint for the variety in the exterior walls, the shapes and materials of the roofs, and the symmetry, coherence, overall appeal, and mellowness of the block. No. 255 Magellan is a slate-roofed, brick house, with gardens on three lots, surrounded by a wrought iron fence, with gilded finial darts.

▪ Next to No. 201 Magellan is a right-of-way that goes to Dewey. Beyond Sola you soon pass the back of the Forest Hill MUNI station. After Plaza you continue to the end of Magellan. Turn left on Castenada to ascend the stairway next to No. 140, a Maybeck-designed house of 1924. The carved grapevines, which symbolize fecundity, along the eaves blend in so well with the surrounding vegetation that you almost fail to see this detail. At the top of the stairs, you're at No. 334 Pacheco. Turn right.

▪ At Alton turn right and then left on Castenada to Ventura. The best weather pattern in Forest Hills is in this northeast section.

▪ No. 2 Castenada, in addition to more recent plantings, has a magnificent, award-winning cactus garden of many varieties, which complement the Southwest style of the house. The owner is augmenting the collection with other varieties of plants.

▪ Turn left on Ventura and ascend the stairway next to No. 60, which continues up to No. 400 Pacheco and No. 70 Alton. The retired resident, to whom I spoke, told me he found great delight in gardening. He said he turns 30-minute gardening tasks into three-hour journeys of the spirit. In the garden in front of the house he has planted marigolds, liatris, red hot poker, pin cushion, honey bush, and some vines. The area sparkles with color. You are at the change-of-name point in the block. Alton begins at No. 70 and continues toward the east. From No. 400 the street becomes Pacheco and runs northwest of the Alton Stairway. How is one to know of these vagaries without getting lost a few times?

- Walk a few feet to the crosswalk to cross the street safely at the Pacheco and Alton street sign. Ascend the 10 steps to upper Pacheco; cross the street to No. 399 Pacheco and continue ascending Alton Stairway.

- At the top of the stairway you are next to No. 60 Sotelo. (To the left at No. 51 is a 1914 Maybeck house with an off-center, octagonal, pulpit-like balcony; the sides are decorated with redwood shingles and an open carved-wood design.) Bear right on Sotelo, then left on 9th Ave. to go right on Mendosa.

- Descend the Montalvo Stairway between Nos. 91 and 99 to upper 9th Ave. Turn right to follow the curve around the planted median and arrive at lower 9th Ave. It's a small price to pay for the aesthetic experience of walking on divided streets.

Pat F. has what, in her southern family, is known as a "bump of direction," that is, a natural, perfect sense of direction.

Pacheco Stairway   *Tony Holiday*

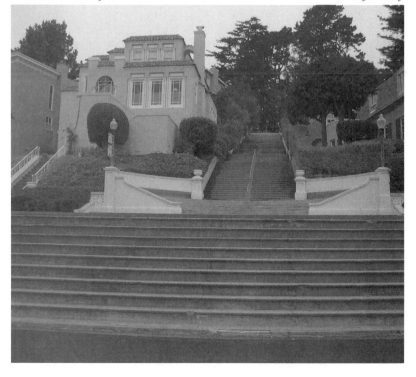

◢ Descend the Montalvo Stairway on lower 9th Ave. (next to No. 2238), past No. 199 San Marcos. You pass a backyard with formal hedges and cobblestone walls and arches. Turn left at Castenada. No. 270, at the corner of Lopez, is another Maybeck home. Built in 1918, it is a three-story, shingled residence with bays and dormers. Next to No. 249 Castenada is the Pacheco Stairway. Descending the grand Pacheco Stairway to the street, I think of Jerry Healy, the first superintendent gardener of the tract (also called the "Mayor of Forest Hill"). Healy planted geraniums and marguerites so that the area was a mass of red and white.

◢ The Maybeck-designed Forest Hill Clubhouse at No. 381 Magellan can be seen by turning right at the bottom of the stairway. Otherwise, descend to Dewey Blvd., to your beginning.

Grading & Sliding,

Forest Knolls

Fog & Drip

Forest Knolls neighborhood is bounded by 7th
Ave. and the Sunset neighborhood on the west,
and by Clarendon and the Twin Peaks neighborhood
to the east. Situated on the south slopes of Mt. Sutro
(918'), it was largely developed for housing in the 1960s.
Though the architecture is similar throughout the curving
streets, the area is rich in geologic history. Over a period of about
10,000 years, alluvial deposits and layers of sand have blown in
from the beach. The terrain can be unstable in times of earthquakes
and heavy rains.

After a landslide occurred in 1966, a 10-year building moratorium
was declared for the area. Beneath the layers of sand, Mt. Sutro is composed mostly of red chert, the dominant rock in the Mt. Davidson and
Twin Peaks area. It accounts for the high elevations in this part of the
City. Chert is one of the hardest components of the Franciscan Formation—little affected by wind and rain—yet it can erode into unstable
clay. Homes built in the 1980s have required expensive engineering to
strengthen them against landslide and earthquake damage.

Adolph Sutro, mayor of San Francisco from 1895 to 1897, loved the
western section of San Francisco. His name is associated with many of
the City's historic legacies: Sutro Baths (Walk 10), Cliff House, Sutro
Library, Sutro Towers, Sutro Forest, Mt. Sutro, and Sutro Heights. Geographically, Forest Knolls was Adolph Sutro's hunting preserve, part
of his fiefdom of one-twelfth of San Francisco. Sutro (1830–1898) a self-
taught mining engineer from Prussia, made his fortune from the sale

of the four-mile tunnel he designed to keep the Comstock silver mines of Nevada operating safely.

In 1995 two footprints were found in a sandy shore of what was once a steep sand dune, now hardened to gray sandstone, along Langebaan Lagoon near Cape Town, South Africa. Discovered by David Roberts, a South African geologist from the Council of Geoscience, they have been identified as the oldest fossilized tracks of an anatomically modern human found to date. They measure about a woman's size-seven shoe and have been dated back 117,000 years.

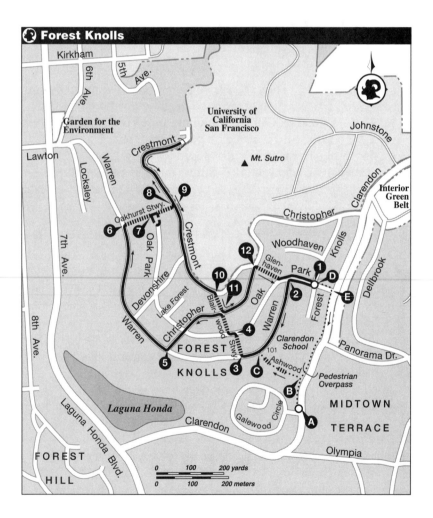

Because the western section of San Francisco receives significant fog, which often settles in treetops, Forest Knolls became a rain forest after Sutro planted thousands of eucalyptus—as well as some Monterey pine and cypress—here and on Twin Peaks, to hold the soil. Sutro established Arbor Day in California during his term as mayor, and schoolchildren participated in planting trees. Today, many of the eucalyptus they planted have been cut or have fallen down. Not only do eucalyptus have a shallow root system, but their life span is a mere century—very brief for a tree. Yet an abundance of trees still provides habitat and food for many birds, including hawks and owls. Trees also

WALK 16 ROUTE: Forest Knolls

Public Transportation: MUNI Bus #36 Teresita. Farther away, several Metro lines stop at Forest Hill Station. For MUNI bus or metro information, call 311 (outside San Francisco call (415) 701-2311).

Note: For those walkers who would like to experience the Ashwood Lane walkway and stairway, begin at the west side of Clarendon, just south of the pillars of the pedestrian overpass at the sign, Galewood Circle, a mini-neighborhood. Begin the walk at A and then continue with B, C, and Step 2.

A. Begin at the Galewood Circle Dr. street sign on the west side of Clarendon.

B. Walk into Ashwood Lane, to the right of Galewood Circle Dr.

C. Continue on the stairway until No. 101 Warren. (Continue with No. 2 below.)

1. Begin at Oak Park and Forest Knolls.

2. Bear left on Warren.

3. Ascend Blairwood Lane Stwy. to Christopher.

4. Bear left on Christopher to Warren.

5. Right on Warren to Oakhurst Stwy (to the left of No. 398 Warren).

6. Ascend Oakhurst Stwy.

7. Right into cul-de-sac of Oak Park and then return to Oakhurst. Right to Crestmont.

8. Detour left on Crestmont, and then return to Oakhurst.

9. Continue on Crestmont to Blairwood Stwy.

10. Descend Blairwood Stwy. to Christopher.

11. Left on Christopher to Glenhaven.

12. Descend Glenhaven Stwy. to Oak Park and your beginning.

D. *Alternate ending:* Walk forward to Clarendon.

E. Right on Clarendon to your beginning.

provide a subtle screening among houses, so look closely to see the edifices on stilts, the birds, the ocean, and the elusive stairways. Residents with whom I've talked express delight in living in a forest, a nonurban section of the City. Yet, a few blocks away they can board MUNI to go to a movie, the library, or the store. Although they receive a disproportionate amount, not once did anyone mention fog. As you walk along here, you'll enjoy breathing the fresh ocean air.

⊿ There's an unusual stairway available to us as a starting point. It's Ashwood Lane Stairway, 0.2 mile from the Oak Park and Forest Knolls beginning, and it illustrates two principles: It provides an important shortcut into the Forest Knolls neighborhood from an important thoroughfare, Clarendon; and the stairway path has the atmosphere of the mountain area that Sutro enjoyed so much. If you do not wish to use this alternate beginning, start your walk at Oak Park and Forest Knolls.

⊿ Continue the walk at Oak Park and Forest Knolls, just off Clarendon. Turn left on Warren. Across from No. 113 Warren is the Blairwood Lane Stairway, which you ascend to Oak Park. Foliose lichen is encrusted on the railings. Lichens flourish where there are no competitive plants and where the air is clean. Vertical gardening is practiced here because of the terrain. I am delighted when I see a successful endeavor. Sedum has been planted on the left among the other vegetation.

⊿ At Oak Park (next to No. 301) cross the street and find a continuation of Blairwood Lane Stairway a few feet to the left. Walk up to Christopher (next to No. 301). The plantings across the street are beautifully terraced with pines, eucalyptus, ice plants, century plants, and marguerites. To the right you can often see fog hanging in the eucalyptus trees on Mt. Sutro.

⊿ Turn left on Christopher. On the slope to the left is a multi-trunked pine covered with lichen. Continue to Warren, and turn right. The attractive single-family dwellings, pastel-colored and angled, thoughtfully allow for maximum light, both reflected and direct.

⊿ Across from No. 399 you ascend what I consider a "floating stairway," the Oakhurst Stairway hidden among eucalyptus. (The *hurst* so often attached to English village names means *wood*.) The hillside on the left has been leveled and drains have been installed. The slope is a sea of emerald green grass in winter. You're in a landscape of eucalyptus, bottlebrush, daisies, weeds, ice plants, and mallow. And the Pacific Ocean extends as far as the eye can see.

◢ The climb is steep. Halfway up the zigzag stairway, you might sit on the steps to admire an extraordinary, wide-angle view as, perhaps, an ocean liner glides east. Finally at Oak Park, you turn right into a narrow walkway that leads into the cul-de-sac. A series of single-family dwellings have been built on your left. Nos. 560 and 550 were built in 1980, the others in 1990 and 1991. I-beams have been driven deep into the rock to provide safety for these homes

Oakhurst Stairway *Peter Nagy*

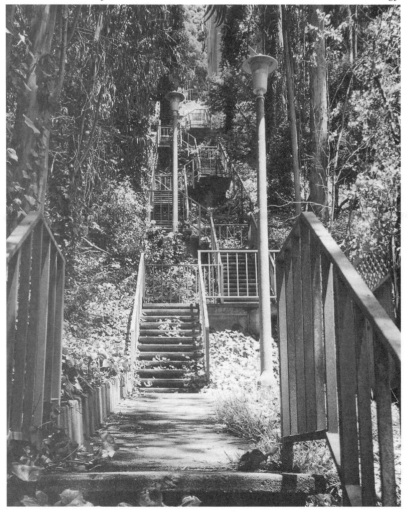

in this landslide area. Return to the stairs and continue your ascent to Crestmont. Orange lichen on the green handrails and blue Vinca major, among the variegated greens of ferns, ivy, and eucalyptus, create visual interest near the long retaining wall ahead, which delineates Sutro Woods, Adolph Sutro's former hunting grounds.

◢ Turn left and explore this part of Forest Knolls before proceeding right. Each house on Crestmont has a garden reached via stairs. Between Nos. 95 and 101, near the white fire hydrant, is the Blairwood Lane Stairway. Descend to Christopher and turn left. Just beyond the Glenhaven Lane Stairway (which you'll descend) next to No. 191, you can see the hillside chert outcropping in colors ranging from beige to red. Now walking down Oak Park, you see a monkey puzzle tree in the distance. Soon you arrive at your beginning.

Further Ambling

Take Clarendon, an important corridor street, to the Twin Peaks, the Forest Hill, or the Golden Gate Heights area. Food is available in the Irving and Judah sections of the Sunset, or the Market and Castro sections of Upper Market. At Lawton and 7th Ave. in the Sunset District, you can explore the Garden for the Environment, a demonstration and teaching site sponsored by Haight Ashbury Neighborhood Council.

Angle

Twin Peaks Foothills

vs. Contour

In the middle of the City is an outcropping of
rock, predominantly composed of chert, basalt,
shale, and sandstone. It was a daunting task to subdi-
vide the area, but short streets and an interconnecting
network of stairways resolved the problem. While the short
streets are in many ways comparable to those on the eastern
side of the City, these hills are higher than either Telegraph Hill
or Russian Hill. The Upper Market neighborhood is known for its
gardens, cooperative neighbors, and attractive, renovated Victorians.

⏹ Begin at Romain and Corbett. Cross Corbett and turn right. As
you pass No. 660 mailbox, you will see a surprise public stairway. However, it leads to a private driveway. Therefore, continue
on Corbett, turn left on Graystone and right onto Copper Alley
Stairway. Descend to Corbett.

⏹ Turn left and continue on Corbett. The views are seen from the
odd-numbered side of the street. Next to No. 555 Corbett is a
framed view of downtown San Francisco. Rooftop Middle School,
Nancy Yoshihara Mayeda Campus, for grades five through eight
is to the left at No. 500. A rock mosaic covers a small portion of the
outside wall with the name Rooftop School. A large mural can be
seen on the inside wall in the playground. Continue past Iron Alley
Stairway at No. 495 Corbett, recently rebuilt and reopened.

⊿ Walk to the intersection of Clayton. For your safety, please use the crosswalks to enter the Neighborhood Garden at the tip of Clayton and Corbett, across the street from the Pemberton Stairway. It is one of the best-designed scraps of land we have. Professional gardeners consider it a gem, and urban explorers are delighted to discover it. In this small space there is much to keep one alert—so many levels and grades to explore and a variety of materials to be sensitive to. Scattered throughout the garden are jade, several varieties of salvia, clematis, black-eyed susan, yellow-and-brown as well as orange irises, and a Norfolk pine.

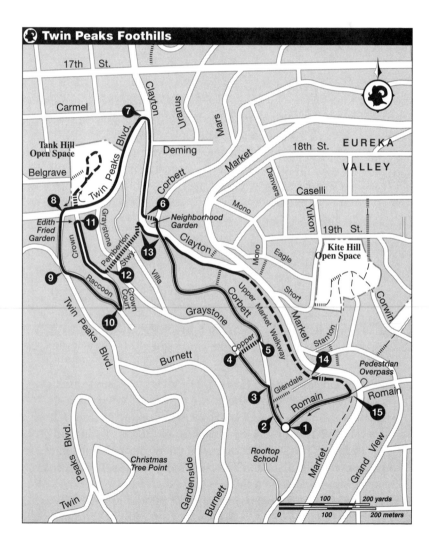

The impact of the Neighborhood Garden is greater than the immediate neighborhood. Over the years, I have seen people in their cars stop, roll down the windows, and thank whoever is working there for the beauty of the garden. The garden has been a volunteer effort since 1960. After the death of Drew Siegal who first transformed the area into a garden, friends have continued to maintain and refine it. Now, one person, Christopher J. Smith, has taken on

WALK 17 ROUTE: Twin Peaks Foothills

Public Transportation: MUNI Bus #37 Corbett. For MUNI bus information, call 311 (outside San Francisco call (415) 701-2311).

1. Begin at Romain and Corbett.
2. Cross Corbett and turn right. Continue to Graystone.
3. Left on Graystone.
4. Right on Copper Alley Stwy. Descend to Corbett.
5. Left on Corbett, past Iron Alley, to Clayton intersection. Cross at crosswalks to corner Neighborhood Garden. Ascend stairway to Clayton.
6. Right on Clayton to Twin Peaks Blvd.
7. Left on Twin Peaks Blvd.
8. Cross Twin Peaks Blvd. and walk up stairway to see view from Tank Hill. Walk around hill and back, descending same stairway, to the boulevard. Turn right to the crosswalk. Turn left and cross the boulevard.
9. Continue on Twin Peaks Blvd., past Mountain Springs, to Raccoon Drive.
10. Bear left on Raccoon Drive to Crown Ct. Sharp left at the bottom of the hill. Walk past No. 127 Crown Ct. and continue on asphalt and stone path to the street. You are now on Crown Terrace.
11. Continue toward end of Crown Terrace. Return to 130 Pemberton Place/98 Crown Terrace across from descending Pemberton Stwy.
12. Descend stairway to Clayton.
13. Right on Clayton. Walk on right side to Market. Continue right onto Upper Market Walkway.
14. Descend and cross Glendale. Ascend stairway to continue on Upper Market Walkway to Romain.
15. Right on Romain to your beginning.

Linking

If you wish to link Twin Peaks Foothills with Upper Market (Walk 18), descend the Pemberton Stwy. to Clayton. Turn left and continue to 17th St. and follow the directions in Walk 18.

You can also link Twin Peaks Foothills with Eureka Valley (Walk 20) to walk other little-known short streets and stairways in the area. To do so, cross Market at the Clayton light. Turn right to descend Mono Stairway to Eagle (Step 10) and follow the directions in Walk 20.

the responsibility for the project. To prevent soil loss on the slope during the rainy season, he has used Sierra stones configured in aesthetic patterns. Although he never thought his degree in theater design would be applied to his new interest in garden design, he has used brick, stone, and concrete judiciously.

- Ascend the stairway to Clayton. Turn right on Clayton and continue to Twin Peaks Blvd. Turn left onto the boulevard and walk on the right sidewalk. Pass Crown Terrace and ascend the short stairway to Tank Hill, one of the last bastions of native wildflowers the City possesses. Again, the interest of one person who has consistently worked to weed and plant on Tank Hill has enriched our lives. You can walk on the covered reservoir installed in 1894 by the Spring Valley Water Company and enjoy an unobstructed view of the City from Lands End on the west to Hunters Point and downtown San Francisco on the east.

If we cross the road, taking care not to be cut down by some rash driver—for they drive at a great pace down these wide streets—we shall find ourselves on top of the hill and beneath shall see the whole of London lying below us. It is a view of perpetual fascination at all hours and in all seasons.

—from *The London Scene* by Virginia Woolf

- Descend the same stairway and turn right. At the pedestrian walk, turn left to cross the boulevard to another beautiful spot where the Edith Fried Garden Association contributes to the maintenance of the Edith Fried Garden. A bench adds another friendly aspect to this small triangle of land in the neighborhood.

- Continue south on Twin Peaks Blvd., past Mountain Springs, to Raccoon Drive and bear left. Raccoon offers a spectacular view, unusual for an access road. Continue down to Crown Court, which is open to vehicles. A few homes are sited on the right. Take a sharp left and walk past No. 127 Crown to No. 125 where you will see the Mt. Diablo range in the East Bay. The stone house on your left (No. 110) is well located in the cul-de-sac. Crown Terrace is part of the district known in the 1930s as Little Italy. The Bank of Italy, subsequently known as Bank of America, held many of the mortgages on the homes (many of which were foreclosed during the Great Depression).

⬛ Continue to the end of Crown Terrace, then return to the intersection signed 130 PEMBERTON PLACE/98 CROWN TERRACE to descend Pemberton Stairway. Continue past Graystone and Villa Terrace to Clayton.

⬛ I enjoy tracking changes in neighborhoods that I have been exploring over a period of years. In 1981 I wrote of that wonderful feeling of luxury I felt the first time I descended the wide section of Pemberton. I thought it was one of the most graceful stairways in the City. The heavy rains of 1982–1983, however, precipitated the deterioration of the brick stairs and the crumbling of the sandstone wall entrance along Clayton. To prevent total collapse, the Department of Public Works installed 4x4 beams.

Pemberton Stairway *Annette Hovie*

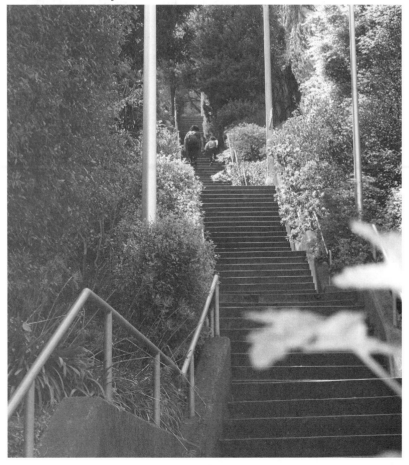

◢ A decade later cooperative work between the residents and the department began. In the year 2000 the defective and dangerous stairs were redesigned according to City code: concrete, but terracotta in color and stamped with a brick-shaped mold. New landscaping was planted: Japanese maples at the landing and shade-tolerant ground covers of Vinca major and jasmine, plus colorful annuals. The last portion to be finished, the wall along Clayton was replaced with an attractive terracotta concrete wall. DPW engineers, landscape architects, and others involved in the Pemberton project enjoyed the challenge of designing a stairway that meets code requirements for safety, as well as the community's aesthetic requirements. The teamwork between the City department and the neighbors began with patient and thorough neighborhood grassroots planning, spearheaded by one of the Pemberton residents. In 2002, a former resident, Rodney Ruskin, presented a drinking fountain in memory of his wife, Myra, and her contributions to the community. It is situated on the Villa Terrace landing.

◢ Turn right on Clayton and walk on the right side to Market. The street sign at the corner reads CLAYTON END & MARKET 3350. Veer right onto the Upper Market Walkway that descends to street level. Cross Glendale and ascend the short stairway back to Upper Market Walkway. Continue to Romain and turn right to your beginning.

Privacy & Quiet

Upper Market

Among the Planets

If you were to walk from Ocean Beach at the western end of the City and finally arrive at 17th St. and Clayton, where this walk begins, you would have worked up to it. The land begins sloping up the eastern side of 19th Ave. At about 4th Ave. and Parnassus, where the University of California is located, the rise is noticeably higher. At 17th St. and Clayton, you're even higher, entering a relatively unknown area where cut-off streets confuse, there is no shopping, and urban walkers relish exploring. A 40-year resident of Upper Terrace says when people realize how difficult it is to maneuver cars on the narrow street, they usually drive away, leaving behind privacy and quiet.

◢ Begin at the intersection of 17th St. and Clayton under the green 17TH STREET 4600 sign. Walk down 17th St. about 50 feet just past the Monument Way Stairway. You can see how the apartment complex is sited on the Franciscan Formation outcrop. Return to ascend the stairway, an abrupt, ambitious beginning, though the rise only extends from 449 to 476 feet. At the top of the stairway you can enjoy an open view of Sutro Forest and the neighborhoods around it, as well as the Marin Headlands, Point Reyes, the Golden Gate Bridge, and Mt. Tamalpais. You're now on Upper Terrace, where multiple dwellings dominate the street.

◢ Turn left on Upper Terrace and walk toward the right of the large, circular, raised-concrete planting area in the middle of the street. In 1887 Adolph Sutro placed the Mt. Olympus monument *Triumph of Light*, a sculpture of a Greek goddess, here to denote the geographical center of San Francisco. If you ascend the stairs, you'll see that the pedestal is still present but the sculpture has been removed. The 360-degree panorama of the City is partially concealed by trees.

> *I love to annotate the phenomena of the city. I can be as solitary in a city street as ever Thoreau was in Walden.*
> —from "Sauntering" by Christopher Morley

◢ Next to No. 480, descend to No. 227 Upper Terrace (lower section). Turn left. Both the quality of the light and the small distinctive

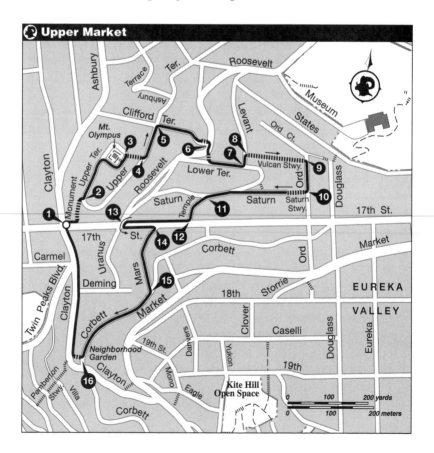

houses contribute to an attractive ambiance. Continue on Upper Terrace to Clifford Terrace. Turn right. At the bottom of the slope, walk down six steps, cross Roosevelt Way to No. 475, and descend the Roosevelt Way Stairway.

◢ Turn left on Lower Terrace to Levant. At the corner, facing one o'clock, you see Corona Heights (Walk 19).

◢ Turn left on Levant and, a few feet away, right onto Vulcan Stairway. A local resident says he knows every step intimately—he used to walk up them daily, all 218 steps. It is a miniature Shangri-la, even though the stairway plantings are overgrown. Neighbors have traditionally worked together to beautify the gardens and walks. On one side of the stairs is a row of remodeled, eclectic,

---

WALK 18 ROUTE: Upper Market

Public Transportation: MUNI Bus #37 Corbett. For MUNI bus and Metro information, call 311 (outside San Francisco call (415) 701-2311).

1. Begin at 17th St. and Clayton. Ascend Monument Way Stwy. to Upper Terrace.
2. Bear left and then right around Mt. Olympus Monument.
3. Next to No. 480 Upper Terrace descend stairway to No. 227 Upper Terrace.
4. Left on Upper Terrace.
5. Right on Clifford Terrace, descend six steps, and cross Roosevelt Way. Next to No. 475 descend stairway to Lower Terrace.
6. Left on Lower Terrace.
7. Left on Levant.
8. Right on Vulcan Stwy. to Ord.
9. Right on Ord to Saturn.
10. Ascend Saturn Stwy. to cul-de-sac. Walk to Temple.
11. Left on Temple.
12. Right on 17th St. to Uranus.
13. Cross 17th St. Left on 17th St. to Mars.
14. Right on Mars, walking on upper level to Corbett.
15. Right on Corbett. Walk on left side to Al's Park. Continue to Clayton.
16. Right at crosswalk into Neighborhood Garden. Ascend stairway to Clayton. Continue right to your beginning.

Linking

If you wish to link Upper Market with Twin Peaks Foothills (Walk 17), complete Walk 18 and then follow directions for Walk 17, Steps 7–15 and then Steps 1–7.

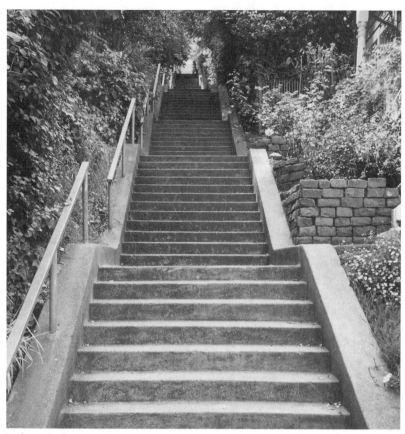

Vulcan Stairway *Peter Nagy*

mostly turn-of-the-century cottages. Well-designed patios and decks extend living outdoors, and skylights open interiors to natural light. English ivy covers the slopes, and in different seasons fuchsia, rhododendron, azaleas, and hydrangeas are in bloom. New residents of the hill to whom I spoke love living here.

At the bottom of Vulcan Stairway at Ord turn right and walk to Saturn Stairway. Visually leading you to the stairway is an area with embedded red bricks on the left and a terraced area with high stone walls to the right. On either side of the center retaining wall and plantings are stairways—one built of railroad ties and the other of concrete. Benches positioned on raised brick and header-board platforms let you sit and enjoy expansive views, while nestled in a garden planted with redwood, acanthus, privet, and agapanthus.

◢ At the top of the stairs you enter a cul-de-sac of Saturn, a divided street where you walk along the upper level where you ascend short stairways on the walkway to Temple. The houses are small.

◢ Turn left on Temple. At 17th St. turn right, heading uphill to Uranus. Cross at the stoplight here, and double-back (left) on 17th St. to Mars. With the 17% grade on this thoroughfare, you can appreciate the difference stairways make in navigating hills. I include a small section on the south side of 17th St. so that you can better appreciate the land contours and also walk by some older homes and cottages, which have been here since the 1880s. This area is part of the Eureka Valley neighborhood, which has one of the oldest functioning community organizations in the City. During the 1980s there was extensive renovation of the Victorian homes here.

◢ Turn right on Mars and walk on the upper side. Continue to Corbett, turn right, and on the left-hand side next to No. 377 is Al's Park, which extends to Market. Al has been taking care of his park for many years and has been most generous in distributing the fruits of his labor. The park contains fountains, flowers, benches, and fruit trees; the apples are wonderful!

◢ Bearing right, you reach Clayton. (In the first decade of the 20th century, this was the site of Mountain House Inn. A wood bridge here covered a water runoff originating from Mountain Spring.) Turn right at the crosswalk and cross to the flourishing Neighborhood Garden (Walk 17) that has been a volunteer effort since 1960.

◢ Ascend the stairway in the garden to Clayton and turn right. Market is below and the Mt. Sutro TV tower is to the left. Don't forget to look back. Continue on Clayton to 17th St. to your beginning. Walk on the right side for Bay views.

Trees, Rocks,

Corona Heights

& Underground Wiring

This walk takes you on both sides of Corona Heights, which is bounded roughly by Roosevelt, 15th St., States, and Castro. From here you have easy access to the neighborhoods south of Market via Castro and Clayton.

The Corona Heights neighborhood walk has the richness and variety of a satisfying meal. The setting is complex. To the west you see the dramatic rock formation of Corona Hill (510'), geologically part of the Franciscan Formation and very near the City's geographical center. To the east you see the hills, the high-rises, and the Bay. Within the neighborhood, you see the shapes and textures of the street trees and individual gardens; the Edwardian houses, ornamented with varied architectural details and painted in appealing color combinations; the small businesses at street level that provide services and goods for everyday needs—laundries, cleaners, coffeehouses, groceries, hardware stores; and a sky unblemished by overhead electrical wires.

⊿ Begin at the intersection of Buena Vista Terrace and Roosevelt Way. Walking downhill on the odd-numbered side of Roosevelt, you face the Bay. Behind you is the large, handsome structure that was St. Joseph's Hospital and is now the 220-unit Park Hill Condominiums.

- Across the street from No. 26 Roosevelt and next to No. 75, which has a tile plaque of the 16th-century fortified tower in Portugal known as Torre de Belem on the right side of the doorway, is the Henry Stairway that you descend to the cul-de-sac. Bottlebrush trees delineate the entrance. Two flat, false-front Italianates—No. 215 (1906) and No. 213 (1905)—and a pitched-roof with a bay at No. 209 (1906) are of particular interest in this block of Henry.

- The hillside continues to be tended by neighbors in the cul-de-sac. To your left is the back of McKinley School, a two-story building. The long and wide trompe l'oeil stairway from the playground up to the classrooms, painted in a variety of colors vertically divided, gives the illusion of a painting. The walls surrounding are decorated with figures, flowers, and words.

- Cross Castro at the stoplight (it's safer) one block to the left at 14th St. There is also a fine corner grocery where you can buy trail nourishment.

- Go back to Henry and turn left. Nos. 195–193 have protruding wires along the porch roof edge to prevent pigeons from roosting there.

- Turn right on Noe. I particularly like this 100 block because it reflects a village ambiance reminiscent of a New York City neighborhood such as Sutton Place. A strong sense of nature pervades the street. The green canopies of ficus, carob, gingko, plane, and eucalyptus, together with the variegated colors of impatiens, fuchsias, daisies, and camellias planted in boxes around small shrubs, create a flourishing environment around the small stores.

- Cross 15th St. and continue to the mini-community garden park at the corner of Noe and Beaver, a felicitous space for friends and neighbors to meet and visit. Turn right on Beaver, where the synergistic effect of a fine assortment of Stick-style Italianates and street trees continues. You are walking uphill. Cross Castro at 16th St. for safer crossing and continue upward on Beaver. There is an attractive, set-back, two-family home and adjoining garden at Nos. 123–125 Beaver (1879). Next to No. 145 Beaver is the DeForest Stairway.

- Before ascending, you may want to look at the unusual wall of chert slickensides across from No. 174 Beaver. As you walk around it (Peixotto Playground is to your right) you see the best example in the City of slickensides, or polished chert. Be sure to rub your hands over the cold, smooth shiny surfaces, the result of millions of years of rock grinding against rock under high pressure.

- Ascend the stairway to the top, where you'll be at the tennis courts of Corona Heights Park.

- Walk through the gate and bear right immediately as you go uphill. Stop for a moment to turn around and look at the Bay, visible between the buildings.

- You are in back of the Randall Museum, commonly known as the Junior Museum. Located at No. 199 Museum Way, it is positioned within one of the most scenic topographical areas in the City—an assemblage of 140-million- to 160-million-year-old chert and sandstone. The Randall Museum is dedicated to Josephine Randall, the first superintendent of recreation in San Francisco. She was able to fulfill her dream of establishing a nature museum to instill in children a love of science, natural history, and the arts. The museum is

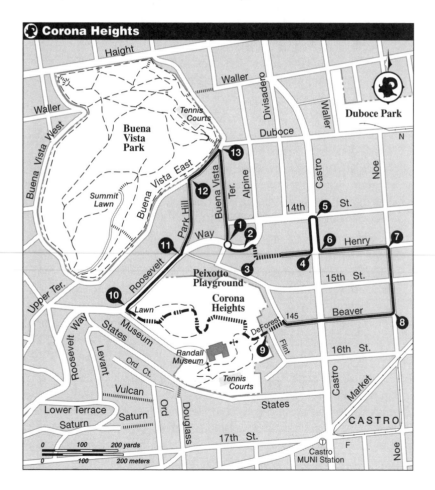

also a popular learning site for adults. It presents lectures; exhibits of geology and anthropology; and classes in natural history, photography, ceramics, and carpentry. It also has an important collection of live native animals, the basis for a popular series of talks. (The museum welcomes volunteers. For more information, call (415) 554-9600.)

⊿ In its present location since 1951, the museum has recently completed several projects: a large deck on the building's east side, new landscaping, and a garden where children are taught the science and art of gardening.

⊿ At the fork in the path where the eucalyptus tree stands, bear right on the stairway. It was installed in 1990 to minimize erosion of the fragile hill and give young native plants an opportunity to take root. Plant-restoration work parties are an ongoing, monthly, volunteer activity. Ahead is a startlingly beautiful panoramic view of the Bay and the hills, downtown San Francisco to the north, and to the south Bernal Heights with its microwave station. You can see McKinley School below to the left, with its striking blue-trimmed vents and red roof. You get a sense of height here, and Corona Hill is a favorite place for rock climbers to practice their skills. A conveniently placed bench is also a perfect station for full-moon viewing.

WALK 19 ROUTE: Corona Heights

Public Transportation: MUNI Bus #37 Corbett. Several Metro Lines stop at the Castro Street Station. For MUNI bus or Metro information, call 311 (outside San Francisco call (415) 701-2311).

1. Begin at Roosevelt Way and Buena Vista Terrace.
2. Walk downhill on odd-numbered side of Roosevelt.
3. Descend Henry Stwy. at No. 473 Roosevelt and continue to Castro.
4. Left to 14th St. Cross Castro.
5. Return back to Henry St.
6. Left on Henry to Noe.
7. Right on Noe to Beaver.
8. Right on Beaver. Next to No. 145 Beaver, ascend DeForest Way Stwy. into Corona Heights Park.
9. Follow path and stairways to Roosevelt.
10. Right on Roosevelt to Park Hill.
11. Left on Park Hill to Buena Vista East.
12. Right on Buena Vista East to Buena Vista Ter.
13. Right on Buena Vista Ter. to your beginning.

To the right at the next landing, the 220-unit Park Hill Condominiums with its distinctive terracotta tile roof can be seen. Continue up the short stairway to the left, and walk to the signpost stating SUMMIT 150 FT. Follow the stairways to the top for a 360-degree view.

In 1881 Dr. Ed Livingstone Trudeau walked the length of Manhattan—from Central Park to the Battery—in 47 minutes on a bet.

From the opposite side of the summit, descend the stairways and path that leads into a clearing adjacent to a dog run. One of the amenities of the dog run is a doggie water fountain. Exit at the gate near the sign that reads RANDALL MUSEUM.

You're at Museum Way and Roosevelt. If you would like to visit the museum, go left on Museum Way for a short distance. The museum, including the gates to the gardens, is open 10 AM to 5 PM Tuesday through Saturday. The walkway to the front entrance is designed with incised replicas of plants and flowers. Inside are traveling and permanent science exhibits. A popular one is the earthquake exhibit, which features a seismograph recording of earthquake action in the area, and the seismometer, which allows you to feel the intensity of a registered earthquake.

McKinley Playground *Adah Bakalinsky*

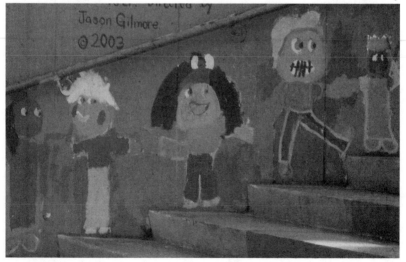

◢ After your visit to the museum return to Roosevelt and turn right. There is an attractive array of varied architecture on this street from the redwood shingle "tuck-in" at No. 284 Roosevelt (1907) to the row of Queen Annes—No. 227 (1900) and Nos. 225 and 223 (1903). The new town houses across the street and farther down are consonant with the ambiance of the block. In addition, the exterior color contributes softness and sparkle to the street.

◢ Continue on Roosevelt to Park Hill and turn left. No. 77 has both a living arbor front door entrance and a living fence.

◢ At Buena Vista East, turn left to see the aesthetic Park Hill condos. The front door and back large glass windows are aligned so that the panoramic view through the back is reflected in the front.

◢ Buena Vista Park, across the street, was designated as a park in 1870, the same year as Golden Gate Park. It has paths, benches, many trees, various elevations, and many wood stairways. It has been undergoing extensive renovation during an erosion-control and reforestation project. (If you have time, amble through now. Otherwise, I heartily recommend you make a special excursion to explore the park.)

◢ Return to the corner of Park Hill to continue on Buena Vista East. No. 181, at the corner of Buena Vista East and Duboce, is an imposing structure on an acre of land with extensive gardens in back. A developer could legally divide the land into five lots. Fortunately, an individual bought the house and lot with the intention of keeping it as a one-family unit. At the grand entrance to the park, turn right on Buena Vista Terrace. Walk past 14th St. to your beginning.

Amazing

Eureka Valley

Footpaths

Eureka Valley encompasses the area below the southeastern slope of Twin Peaks. Wedged between Diamond Heights, Noe Valley, and Upper Market, it has one of the oldest, continuously functioning neighborhood associations in the City. In the 1920s, the composition of the neighborhood was Scandinavian and Irish. The Swedish church was on Dolores St.; the Scandinavian deli on Market. John Nurmi's bar at No. 258 Noe was a great gathering place for the Finnish residents. Schubert's Bakery employed 10 bakers and was famous citywide for its excellent pastries.

The bakery was the reason that Joseph Affolter's father moved his butcher shop to No. 2283 Market in 1930—he wanted the overflow of customers from the bakery. After he retired, four sons operated the butcher shop for more than 50 years until their deaths. The sign on the wall said, DON'T SWEAR. SMILE. When I spoke to him, Joseph recalled that all the meat, including the beef stew, was sold with bone in it, and the fillet was part of the sirloin and tenderloin cuts. Families used to shop twice a day for meat and fish.

Eureka Valley's Castro St. (now known as the Castro neighborhood) is the shopping center and hub of the gay community, an important sociological and political force in San Francisco since 1970. In 1977, Harvey Milk became the first openly gay member of the San Francisco Board of Supervisors. (His photography shop and campaign headquarters at Nos. 573–575 Castro is now City Landmark No. 227.) Milk and Mayor George Moscone were murdered in City

Hall in November 1978 by Dan White, a deranged former supervisor. Harry Britt was appointed to Milk's former position as an openly gay supervisor. The gay movement's militancy created an awareness in the general public of discrimination against gays and lesbians in the police department and in the workplace; it was also effective in influencing the Board of Supervisors to pass the San Francisco domestic partners law, which provides health insurance benefits for partners of gay City employees.

Castro supports a variety of boutiques, stores, restaurants, and bars. The crown jewel of the street is the historic landmark Castro Theatre. Their programming includes revivals of American and foreign films and special events such as the Lesbian and Gay Film Festival, the Jewish Film Festival, and the Silent Film Festival. Every evening an organist plays the Wurlitzer before the first show. He also accompanies silent features. Timothy Pfleuger designed the 1922 Spanish Renaissance–style movie palace, as well as the former Pacific Exchange (now an Equinox Fitness Center), 450 Sutter Building, and the Paramount Theatre in Oakland. The gay influence is apparent in many facets of street life—the rainbow banners attached to the light standards; the many skillful renovations of Victorian homes throughout the neighborhood; the generally available taxis because of the abundance of street traffic; people carrying bouquets of flowers—as gifts or for their homes; the Twin Peaks Tavern at Market, an enduring and highly visible presence for more than 30 years; and the popular Cliff's Hardware, which is one of the best in San Francisco.

The Eureka Valley walk is a favorite of mine. More strenuous than some, it has an eloquent cadence of many kinds of stairways; paths, alleyways, and skyways; unusual gardens; tree-lined streets; open spaces; and houses with special architectural details. The area maintains visual interest through many repeated strolls. Views from it are exceptional. Bring binoculars and perhaps an orange or two (for greater energy).

◢ Begin at Elizabeth and Douglass and walk west on the right-hand side of Elizabeth. You are gradually walking uphill—a perfect introduction to the sidewalk stairway that begins at Hoffman. Abundant and diverse vegetation grows on both sides of the street. Several homeowners decided to put in garages on Elizabeth that cut into the previously long, uninterrupted stairway. The residents of No. 966 display a garden of disarming combinations of colors and textures. After crossing Grand View, bear right to the

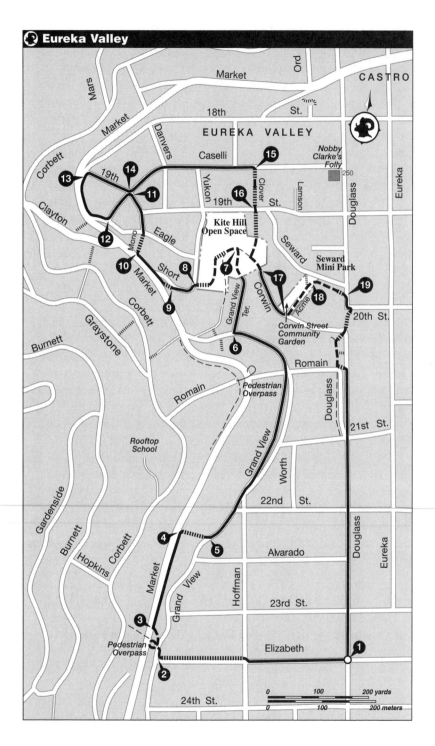

pedestrian overpass above Market, where you have a wondrous view of the eastern half of the City.

⊿ Turn right on Market. At No. 3801 turn right onto the Dixie Stairway, and descend to Grand View.

⊿ Continue to the left on Grand View. At 22nd St., walk on the left side on upper Grand View where you'll see a curly leaf willow growing here. Walk past Romain along this divided street.

WALK 20 ROUTE: Eureka Valley

Public Transportation: MUNI Bus #48 Quintara, #24 Divisadero. For MUNI bus information, call 311 (outside San Francisco call (415) 701-2311).

1. Begin at Elizabeth and Douglass. Walk one block on the right-hand side of Elizabeth to Hoffman. Ascend the sidewalk stairway to Grand View.
2. Cross Grand View and walk on pedestrian overpass to Market.
3. Right on Market.
4. Right on Dixie Stwy. (next to No. 3801 Market) to Grand View (across from No. 285).
5. Left on Grand View. Continue on upper side to Grand View Terrace.
6. Right on Grand View Terrace to enter Kite Hill Open Space.
7. Bear left on second footpath and railroad-tie stairway down to Yukon between Short and Eagle.
8. Left on Yukon to Short. Bear right and ascend Short Stwy. to Market.
9. Right on Market.
10. Right on Mono Stwy. to Eagle. Cross Eagle to continue on Mono right-of-way to 19th St.
11. Veer left on 19th St. to Caselli. Left on Caselli.
12. Right on Eagle to Market. Turn right onto Market.
13. Right on 19th St., facing Kite Hill.
14. Left on Caselli.
15. Next to No. 101 Caselli, ascend Clover Lane Stwy. to 19th St.
16. Cross 19th St. and continue up the stairway, next to No. 4615, onto a dirt path on the north side of Kite Hill.
17. Follow the left path leading into Corwin and walk to Corwin Street Community Garden on the left side of the street opposite No. 95; walk down the (Acme Alley) driveway beside the garden to Seward Mini Park opposite No. 30 Seward.
18. Right on upper pedestrian walkway of Seward. Descend stairway to Douglass.
19. Right on Douglass to 20th. Ascend Douglass Stwy. Cross Corwin and ascend stairway. Walk on pedestrian walkway of Douglass (right side) to Romain. Descend stairway and continue on Douglass to Elizabeth, to your beginning.

- Make a right turn on Grand View Terrace, which leads to Kite Hill Open Space. Purchased with Open Space funds, Kite Hill is inviting and functional. Walkers use it, as do dogs and their owners. While sitting on a bench here, I overheard a lengthy discussion among dog owners about dog personality types, while their pets were enjoying playtime.

- On the Yukon slope of Kite Hill (toward 19th St.), the Natural Areas Program of the Recreation and Park Department has restored native plants that once grew here. I saw among them: gooseberry (*Ribes*), footsteps of spring (*Sanicula arctopoides*), wild parsley (*Lomatium dasycarpum*), a favorite of the anise swallowtail butterfly, California buttercup (*Ranunculus californicus*), California aster (*Aster chilensis*), and California brome grass (*Bromus californica*). From the top of the hill there's a triangular configuration of Open Space areas: Tank Hill to the left, Corona Heights to the right, and Kite Hill, where you stand at the apex. At the corner of Yukon and 19th St., at the base of the Open Space area, a resident planted a flourishing garden of ginger, echium, and euphorbia, which is counter to the overall native-species restoration of this area.

- Bear left on the second footpath and railroad-tie stairway to Yukon between Eagle and Short. Turn left, walk across to Short, bear right, and continue past valerian and nasturtium growing along the retaining wall. Ascend Short Stairway to Market, turn right, and continue to Mono Stairway.

- Turn right on Mono Stairway to Eagle. Growing alongside are lantana, ceanothus, and rock rose, which has white petals with red targets, indicating the route to the nectar. Cross Eagle to continue to 19th St. on the Mono right-of-way, with its "archaeological" paving mix, consisting of new and old brick, and concrete. Here, at the end of Mono, a neighbor has turned an unused city lot into a veritable Shangri-la. The David Austin roses not only look magnificent, but their aroma is heavenly. At least 30 varieties of birds come here to feed and sing. I was rooted to the spot.

- Turn left on 19th St. and left again onto Caselli. Near No. 312 Caselli the street is edged with cobblestone.

- Turn right on Eagle and right on Market, originally Falcon Road, and later transformed into a toll road named Corbett. Market did not exist west of Eureka until the 1920s. Yet, between 1956 and 1958 it was widened to four lanes. Usually Market is a thoroughfare you drive, so walking here reveals a trove of unsuspected architecture and gardens.

◢ On the hill across the street, at No. 3224, is a large pink house (two smaller ones are later additions) on a 90-foot-deep lot. Known as the Miller-Joost House, it was built in 1867 by Adam Miller, German immigrant, carpenter, and dairy rancher. The house was later occupied by Miller's daughter and her husband, Behrend Joost, who built the first electric railroad from Steuart and Market to the county line in Colma. He also owned the local Mountain Springs Water Co., until the Twin Peaks Tunnel excavation disrupted the flow. The Miller-Joost House has landmark status (Landmark 79). (If this piques your interest, see "Further Ambling" at the end of this walk.) One of my favorite murals by Betsie Miller-Kusz is on the wall next to it. I call it the "Landscape of San Francisco."

◢ Turn right on 19th St., where you will be facing Kite Hill. Turn left on Caselli. At the corner of Danvers, a former church is now a private home.

◢ Next to No. 101 Caselli, on the right side of the street, ascend the Clover Lane Stairway to 19th St. The walkway here is reminiscent of an old-fashioned alley in Chicago. Near No. 4612 19th St. (top of stairway) cross the street and continue up the stairway beside No. 4615. The dirt section above this stairway leads to the north side of Kite Hill. A bench located here is perfect for contemplating the 135-degree view of the Bay Bridge. Walk to your left to take in a view of Corona Heights and the downtown skyline, with Eureka Valley and the U.S. Mint in the foreground.

◢ From the bench, follow the path right branching into Corwin. Across the street is the remarkable Corwin Street Community Garden. I've been fortunate to have seen the metamorphosis of this section of land. The signage is excellent; the choice of vegetation is botanically superior; butterflies and birds use this garden and in return, pollinate and sing. Among the beds of 67 native flowers, shrubs, and trees attractive to butterflies and hummingbirds are yarrow, mimulus, coyote bush, and mallow.

Mary Walker, 82, of Philadelphia became a walker during a transit strike. For years, she had held down a full-time job at one of the nation's largest banks. After work each day, she put on her sneakers and took the 7.5-mile walk home. She enjoyed every bit of the walk and saw people racing by, which was not her style. As she explained, "I get home when I get home."

- Walk down the condo driveway, Acme Alley, next to the garden entrance to Seward Mini Park. With the added benefit of being protected from wind, it's a fine setting for a picnic lunch. In the early days of San Francisco, Acme Alley was the path used to take cattle from Mission Dolores to pasture.

- Turn right on upper Seward. This elevated pedestrian walkway gives you a better view of neighborhood gardens. Continue on this walkway and descend the stairway to Douglass.

- Turn right to 20th St. and right to ascend the Douglass Stairway. At the top, look back at the view of Corona Heights Hill. Cross Corwin and ascend the stairway to the upper level of divided Douglass to enjoy a better view.

- Descend the stairway at Romain to Douglass. The Alvarado Elementary School at No. 625 Douglass (at the corner of 22nd St.) has a mural flanking the school entrance, in memory of two wonderful teachers. Through the initiative and leadership of sculptor Ruth Asawa, the school has had an enrichment art program for the past 42 years. Asawa has used children's art for her public fountains in the Hyatt Hotel courtyard and in Ghirardelli Square. Her son and daughter have continued the Asawa family tradition which has become a community legacy.

- The school walls and fence are painted with city scenes and water scenes. One section of the fence is decorated with painted mosaic tiles of a school, a bus, and children's heads in a tree. Assembled on the outer side of a wall of the playground is a 42 x 11-foot ceramic mural with a theme of nature and gardening dedicated to Ruth Asawa. It was completed in May 2000, a two-year project in which students, teachers, and artists participated. In 2010, the School of the Arts High School was renamed the Ruth Asawa San Francisco School of Arts.

- At the corner of 23rd St. are five false-gable, rectangular-bay homes to your left. From the middle of the street looking west (in line with the middle of Twin Peaks), you might recall Daniel Burnham's plan for a magnificent viewing corridor from the Ferry Bldg. to Twin Peaks. The 1906 earthquake, and subsequent hurried rebuilding, prevented his 1905 San Francisco City Beautiful plan from being implemented.

- Continue to Elizabeth to your beginning.

Further Ambling

"Nobby" Clarke's Folly at No. 250 Douglass (at the corner of Caselli) is a king-sized Queen Anne mansion with landmark status. Built on a 17-acre lot in 1892 for $100,000, it was composed of 5 stories, 45 rooms, 52 closets, 10 fireplaces, and 272 windows. The mansion has since been converted to 15 one-bedroom apartments.

Clarke was an Irish sailor who immigrated to California in 1850. Beginning his career as a gold miner, he later worked in the police department, became a lawyer and, finally, pursued a career as an entrepreneur. The springs flowing from Joost's property in upper Twin Peaks followed the north side of Caselli to Clarke's holdings. Becoming dissatisfied with the service, he started Clarke's Water Works, but in 1896 he went bankrupt.

A Mondrian

Dolores Heights

Walk

A good walk is an organism of mysterious nuances that can affect us in subtle ways, from quiet harmoniousness to ebullience, from languor to exuberance. Within a stroll for a stamp, a loaf of bread, a bit of exercise, or a breath of fresh air are the promising ingredients of an imaginative walk that charms and delights: the various terrain to step over, the spectrum of sky colors to see, the views of manufactured objects to comprehend, the assortment of people to meet, and the intrinsic rhythm and shape of the walk to sense.

I love to trace out the shape of a walk on paper after I walk it. I want to know if there is a correlation between the shape and how it feels when I walk. There is! For some reason that I don't understand, my early walks usually traced into the shape of a foot or a shoe, and the walks felt very comfortable. Now my walks seem to form fanciful figures, or geometric, Piet Mondrian configurations, and they feel effortless. The Dolores Heights walk is Mondrian choreography!

◢ Begin at 19th St. and Sanchez. Ceanothus, bottlebrush, and acacia grow at the base of the imposing wall flanking the double stairways going up Sanchez. (The first City inspection is recorded on the stairways in 1939.) I ascend the left stairway. A contemporary home at the top, No. 615 Sanchez, has replaced a small house that once stood here. The four cypress trees in front of the house are more than 50 years old. At one time Sanchez had brick paving, but it was too slick and had to be covered with asphalt.

◢ Approaching the intersection of Cumberland and Sanchez, I am impressed that this is still one of my favorite corners in San Francisco. What makes me feel this is the combination of houses and trees, a feeling of neighborliness that pervades the street, the configuration of the two streets affording both close-up and distant views, and the surprise of seeing all this at the end of the first ascent of this route.

◢ Continue walking on Sanchez. A few feet farther on, you can see the section of the Cumberland Stairway that goes down to Church. At No. 650 Sanchez (at Cumberland) Cape jasmine and trumpet vine grow under the veranda. Penstemon, valerian, mimulus, rosemary, and acanthus brighten the block. Continue walking on the left (east) side of Sanchez. At Cumberland, the dome of the Christian Science Temple on Dolores is visible.

◢ In front of No. 655 Sanchez, descend the stairs to the pedestrian walkway. Go to your right. At No. 674 Sanchez, New Zealand flax grows behind the rock. You're walking south toward 20th St. on the east side of the street. A center strip of flora and unusual tilted stairs divide the upper and lower parts of Sanchez between 20th St. and Liberty. Continue walking on the left side of lower Sanchez. Ascend the stairway to Liberty.

Cumberland Stairway   *Tony Holiday*

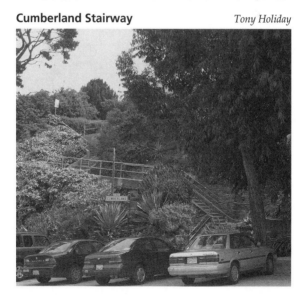

◢ Cross Liberty to continue up the Sanchez Stairway, which is fronted by a high retaining wall. The redwood-shingled house, No. 746 Sanchez, conforms to the irregular-shaped lot in a comfortable way; it stretches around the corner. The off-center, arched veranda or possibly carport (although there is a garage off to the side) leads the eye to the terraced garden, where camellias and a mature Douglas-fir are the dominant plants.

◢ Continue to 21st St. The house at the corner, No. 3690, formerly belonged to James "Sunny Jim" Rolph, Jr., the popular San Francisco mayor (1912–1931). John McLaren, who was the superintendent of Golden Gate Park for 60 years, planted the Monterey pine trees around the house. At No. 3701 21st St., a sculptured redwood bench is inset on tile and dedicated to Audrey Penn Rodgers by friends, relatives, and neighbors. She was president of the

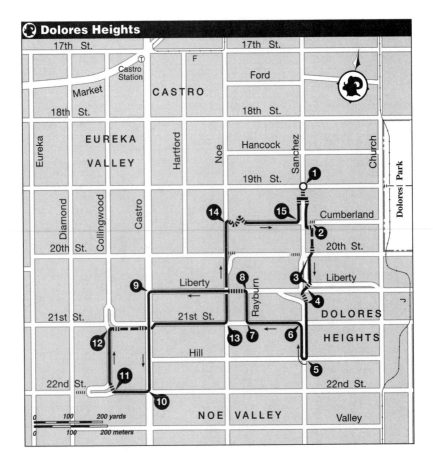

Dolores Heights Improvement Club for many years and diligently watched over the area to make sure it retained its unique neighborhood ambiance.

The swiftest traveler is he that goes afoot.

—Henry David Thoreau

⬛ Walk toward Hill, formerly called "nanny goat hill" in reference to the goats that grazed here, and enjoy the view to the south. At the turn of the century, the designated neighborhood voting place was a small structure on the top of the hill (right). Before the streets were paved, firefighters, who worked at the 22nd St. firehouse between Sanchez and Noe (now a residence), left their pumps up here on the hill as a kindness to their horses.

⬛ With so many springs in the area, the Native Americans who once lived near Mission Dolores came up here to get their water. There are still some houses in the neighborhood that have their own capped wells.

WALK 21 ROUTE: Dolores Heights

Public Transportation: MUNI Bus #33 Stanyan; Metro J Church. For MUNI bus or Metro information, call 311 (outside San Francisco call (415) 701-2311).

1. Begin at 19th St. and Sanchez. Ascend Sanchez Stwy. to Cumberland.
2. At No. 655 Sanchez descend small stairway. Turn right onto pedestrian walkway to 20th St.
3. Continue on left side onto lower Sanchez. Ascend stairway to Liberty.
4. Cross Liberty to ascend Sanchez Stwy. Continue past 21st St. to Hill St.
5. Loop back on Sanchez to 21st St.
6. Left on 21st St. to Rayburn.
7. Right on Rayburn to Liberty.
8. Left on Liberty. Descend stairway to Noe. Continue to Castro.
9. Left on Castro to 22nd St.
10. Right on 22nd St.
11. Right and ascend stairway to Collingwood. Walk to 21st St.
12. Right on 21st St. Descend sidewalk stairway. Continue past Castro to Noe.
13. Left on Noe to Cumberland Stwy. across from No. 670 Noe.
14. Right to ascend Cumberland Stwy. Continue to Sanchez.
15. Left on Sanchez. Descend Sanchez Stwy. to 19th St. to your beginning.

- Historically, working-class people have resided in Dolores Heights, but now many professional people live here, and the mix enriches the neighborhood. The residents love the sunny, fog-free weather.

- At Hill and Sanchez look left to take the full measure of the elevation. Retrace your steps on Sanchez to 21st St. and turn left. Turn right on Rayburn, which takes you out to Liberty. After a left turn, you soon reach the Liberty Stairway, which you descend to Noe.

- Four, white, stucco Art Deco houses alongside the stairway are foils for the multitude of neighborhood Victorians, from elaborate Queen Annes of the late 1880s and 1890s to one-story, flat-front Italianates of the 1870s and early 1880s.

- Walking in the neighborhood, I was captivated by the constantly shifting cloud cover playing with the TV tower on Mt. Sutro, obscuring it one minute and uncovering it the next. Be flexible about crossing the street for better views.

- Cross Noe. Walk on the left (south) side of Liberty. The 500 block of Liberty is exquisite, with small and mature trees—plane, magnolia, and Brisbane box. Nos. 564–576 Liberty were built in 1897 by Fernando Nelson, a prolific developer of tract Victorians in this and other Mission neighborhoods. These houses display his favorite wood embellishments: the decorative circles and pendants that he styled "donuts" and "drips."

- Continue on Liberty to Castro. Corona Heights comes into view. Turn left on Castro. Queen Anne row houses are on the even-number side of the 700 block of Castro. (Look for the donuts and drips.)

- Walk to 22nd St. and turn right. This section of 22nd St. is a turnabout; a sculptural, high-curved retaining wall encompasses the stairway you now ascend to Collingwood. (The stairway beyond it goes down to Diamond.) You're at the top of the hill of this five-block-long street.

- Turn right on Collingwood. In 1932, a German mason built the cobblestone house at No. 480, using stones from the dismantled Castro cable car line. Turn right on 21st St., which used to be extremely steep from Diamond to Castro. In 1924 the City "improved" the street by lowering the grade on one side while raising it on the other, resulting in a grade-separated street and some nonfunctioning garages. The one at No. 3937 was converted into living space.

- Walk down the sidewalk stairway on the odd-numbered side of 21st St. and continue to Noe. The 3800 block of 21st St. has an exceptional row of Queen Anne Victorians. On the left side, they gently follow the slope of the hill. John Anderson, a contractor, built Nos. 3836–3616 in 1903 and 1904. Your view from here includes the top third of the TV tower.

◢ Turn left on Noe. At Liberty, look right to see the stairway you have previously descended. From No. 741 (on the odd-numbered side of Noe), you can see the skyline to the north and west. Continue on Noe past the curved retaining wall of 20th St. and the narrow stairway alongside the apartment house at No. 695. The houses on the even-numbered side of the street have the potential to become a showcase like those on Alamo Square, or on Clay across from Alta Plaza Park. Three-quarters of the ubiquitous Mt. Sutro TV Tower is still in sight.

◢ Ascend the Cumberland Stairway across from No. 670 Noe. The retaining wall, made from cobblestones, is a backdrop to the rock outcropping upon which the stairway was built. Several century plants, set into the rock soil, form a strong upright profile against the jumbled Franciscan Formation. Sedum, gazanias, and ivy grow here and there.

◢ From the cul-de-sac entrance at the top of the stairs, begin a pleasant walk alongside tree-lined houses. The Dolores Heights Special Use District, which runs from Cumberland to part of 22nd St. between Noe and Church, was established in 1980 to provide residential-design guidelines and preserve front gardens. No. 367 has an octagonal belvedere, roofed in a pattern of blue and lavender tiles. On the cobblestone terrace of No. 338 Cumberland, goldfish swim in the pond. The exterior of No. 333 is cement composition board, a relatively new material being used in San Francisco. The house provides contrast and a contemporary link to the Victorian architecture in the neighborhood. No. 332 is a simple Craftsman-style house. No. 300 is made up of two 1906 refugee cottages, which were originally located in Dolores Park. Known as bonus-plan cottages, they provided affordable housing to those who lost their homes in the 1906 earthquake and fire. (The Finance Relief, the Red Cross, and the U.S. Army originally funded the project.) The Carpenters Union, Local 22, built 5,610 shacks. In 1997, 17 shacks were still extant.

◢ Continue to Sanchez to arrive at my favorite corner of Cumberland. Turn left and descend the Sanchez Stairway to your beginning. Places to eat are plentiful along Castro, 18th St., and Market.

From Ship Building

Potrero Hill

Through Dot-Com

to Biotech

Geographically, the Potrero Hill neighborhood is
bound by 16th St. to the north, Cesar Chavez to the
south, Potrero Ave. to the west, and San Francisco Bay
to the east. Highway 101 to the west and Highway 280 to
the east are additional nearby boundaries that provide easy
access to and from other parts of the City. Geologically, Potrero
Hill is composed mainly of serpentine rock. At 300', it commands
encompassing views of the City. Climatically, Potrero Hill has some
of the best weather in San Francisco because the larger hills to the west
shelter it from winds. Sociologically, it is known for its strong sense of
community, and its ethnically and racially diverse population.

When the Spaniards arrived in the 18th century, the Potrero Hill
area was a peninsula with its original shoreline intact. It was also pasture land (*potrero* means *pasture* in Spanish). Horses, cows, and goats
grazed the hill during the Spanish and Mexican period. In the latter
half of the 19th century, industry located here because of the proximity to water. Union Iron Works was one of the largest builders of steel
steamships and men-of-war. It later became Bethlehem-Todd. Baker
and Hamilton's warehouse was here in 1849; the site is now occupied
by Show Place Square and the Galleria Design Center. Tubbs Cordage
was in business in 1859, and Tubbs St. is listed on the maps.

Workers for these industries came from Ireland, Scotland, and the Balkans. Irish Hill was located at 22nd St. and Illinois; Scottish shipbuilders mostly lived on Connecticut. In the early 1900s, Greeks and immigrants from Eastern Europe seemed to congregate near Mariposa and Vermont. Molokans, a religious sect predominantly composed of Russian peasants who, in the 1550s, rejected czarist church policy and beliefs of orthodox Christians, settled around Carolina near 20th St. (No. 341 Carolina). Boardinghouses for workers were along Illinois and 3rd St.; cottages along Tennessee cost $585.

Because Potrero Hill was unscathed by the 1906 earthquake and fire, people from destroyed areas migrated here. The tent city, official Relief Camp No. 10, extended north to Mariposa, south to between 20th and 22nd Sts., west to Indiana, and east to Kentucky (now 3rd St.). In March 1907 the tents could be exchanged for cottages at a cost of $6 per month. Renters could move the cottages to their own lots. Good weather, good transportation, good views in every direction, and available lots at good prices attracted professionals and artists to the area after World War II. Cooperative community spirit is responsible for the plethora of community gardens, social services available for the elderly and children, and for resolution of long-term environmental problems such as air pollution from the Pacific Gas & Electric power plants. By the end of 2010, the last operating power plant will shut down. Trans Bay Cable now provides the City with a new source of electricity from the town of Pittsburg in the East Bay without having to install a power generation plant in San Francisco.

◢ The walk begins in front of the Potrero Hill Neighborhood House (commonly called NABE, pronounced with a long A) at 953 De Haro at Southern Heights. It was founded in 1907 by the Presbyterian Church Women's Group to help immigrant groups learn English and cope with changes in their everyday lives. Since 1922, it has been located in architect Julia Morgan's Craftsman-style landmark building (No. 86).

◢ NABE continues in the spirit of Jane Addams' Hull House in Chicago and Neighborhood House in St. Paul (my second home while I was growing up) in its relationship to the community. In addition to the array of activities available, including Head Start classes, senior lunches and socializing, and art and drama classes for young people, NABE is everybody's wonderful grandfather, an understanding listener, a protective and caring mentor. The legendary Enola Maxwell was the director of NABE from 1972 until her death in 2004. Her grandson, Edward Hatter, is the current director. *The Potrero View*, the community newspaper, rents office space in NABE. Ruth Passen was the volunteer editor for 37 years. Steve Moss is the current publisher and editor.

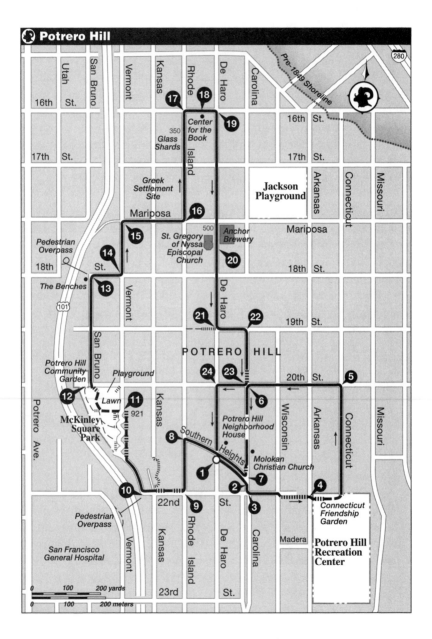

◢ NABE is both the beginning of and the pivotal point in your walk. From here you have a continuous view in every direction. Orient yourself before proceeding on the walk: To the north you have a close-up view of the downtown skyline; east, the Bay Bridge and Yerba Buena Island; south, Candlestick Hill; southwest, San Francisco General Hospital; and west, Twin Peaks.

WALK 22 ROUTE: Potrero Hill

Public Transportation: MUNI Bus #19 Polk; #22 Fillmore; #10 Townsend; #48 Quintara. For MUNI bus information, call 311 (outside San Francisco call (415) 701-2311).

1. Begin at De Haro and Southern Heights (from Portrero Hill Neighborhood House, or NABE, at 953 De Haro).
2. Walk southeast on curve of Southern Heights to 22nd St.
3. Left on 22nd and descend 22nd St. Stwy. to Arkansas.
4. Cross Arkansas and descend stairway. Continue on path to Connecticut. Left on Connecticut to 20th St.
5. Left on 20th to Carolina.
6. Left on Carolina. Continue to ascend short stairway onto Southern Heights.
7. Curve right on Southern Heights to Rhode Island.
8. Left on Rhode Island to 22nd.
9. Right on 22nd and descend 22nd St. Stwy. Bear right past Kansas to Vermont.
10. Right on Vermont. At No. 921 Vermont turn right and ascend stairway. At top of stairway, cross Vermont into McKinley Square Park.
11. Bear left on path around park (past play area). Descend stairway at corner of San Bruno and 20th St.
12. Cross street and walk along San Bruno to 18th St.
13. Right on 18th St. to Vermont.
14. Left on Vermont to Mariposa.
15. Right on Mariposa to Rhode Island.
16. Left on Rhode Island to No. 350.
17. Walk on Rhode Island to 16th St. Right on 16th St.
18. Continue past San Francisco Center for the Book to De Haro.
19. Right on De Haro past St. Gregory of Nyssa Episcopal Church at No. 500.
20. Continue on De Haro to 19th St.
21. Left on 19th St. to Carolina.
22. Right on Carolina. Ascend stairway to 20th St.
23. Right on 20th St. to De Haro.
24. Left on De Haro to your beginning.

◢ From NABE on De Haro, walk southeast along Southern Heights, curving left to 22nd St., at the crest of the hill. Among the foliage in the area is a Norfolk Island pine. Turning left on 22nd St., you pass a water reservoir built on an arresting serpentine rock formation. Descend 22nd St. Stairway to Arkansas. This stairway is a pleasure to traverse because the proportion of riser to tread is exquisite. To the left of the stairway is a rocky area. Fennel grows well here, but it's impossible to use this area for a garden. At the bottom of the stairway, we are on Arkansas. I not only find it pleasing to the eye but conducive to imagining being a neighbor. Along this street and neighboring streets there are a variety of trees from magnolia to ficus and passion flower vines.

◢ Cross the street and turn slightly to the right where you will descend a wood plank stairway adjacent to the Connecticut Friendship Garden. In this area is a buckeye tree and coyote brush. Continue on the dirt path to Connecticut. The gate is on Connecticut, and if someone is working there, you may be able to enter. The small annual flower garden to the left of the poles may be an extension of the garden. To the right is the Potrero Hill Recreation Center.

◢ Turn left on Connecticut. The architectural and botanical mix includes several Stick-style homes built in the 1880s (Nos. 524–512) and a variety of street trees, such as jacaranda, ficus, and Victorian box.

◢ Turn left on 20th St. The Potrero Branch Library across the street at 1616 20th St. has a neighborhood archive collection, popular reading programs for children, and lectures for adults.

◢ At Wisconsin you will see palms, ferns, and fuschia. Continue to Carolina and turn left. Walk on the right side of the street in order to better view the large serpentine outcropping upon which structures have been built. When you're almost opposite the Molokan Christian Church, walk up the stairway.

◢ When you reach Southern Heights, turn right, as it curves to Rhode Island. Turn left on Rhode Island. As you walk downhill, you will notice, on the right, a cottage situated near the back of the lots, known as a "tuck-in." This particular one was built around 1910. On the left, houses are built high on the hill. Next to No. 949, you can see the radio antennae on San Bruno Mountain. Bernal Heights, with its antiquated microwave station, is on the rise to the right of the mountain. Silhouettes of the hills are clearly delineated.

◢ Turn right on 22nd St. Go down the short, steep 22nd St. (sidewalk) Stairway. Pass Kansas, and bear right on Vermont. On the slope to your right, agave, morning glory, and cypress trees are growing. A sound wall on the left mitigates some of the heavy traffic noise of Highway 101.

◢ Walk up Vermont and ascend the stairway on the right in front of the houses into McKinley Square Park.

William Wordsworth walked 14 miles a day in his beloved English Lake District, and an estimated 185,000 miles in his lifetime.

◢ Curve around the walkway to the left. You will see swirls of steam from the San Francisco General Hospital laundry facility. When I was there, a gentleman was reading at the redwood table under the cypress, and dogs and their owners were using the designated dog run. Renovated and redesigned by landscape architect John Thomas, the park was dedicated in September 1999. When the mayor gave the signal, a group of neighborhood children snipped the official ribbon. The new playground is colorful and attractive to children who enjoy exploring the various shapes of play equipment. New benches are very convenient for picnicking and enjoying views, which give youngsters a great opportunity to identify City landmarks.

◢ Beyond the play area, you descend the short stairway to the corner of San Bruno and 20th St. Here on top of the low retaining wall along the sidewalk is a brass U.S. Geodetic Survey reference mark, which was placed here in 1932. At San Bruno and 20th St., cross the street and walk along San Bruno to look at the flourishing Potrero Hill Community Garden.

◢ Continue on San Bruno. Sunbursts adorn the three gables on Nos. 713–715. The block has flat-front Italianates, many of them redone with "misguided improvements," as architectural historian Judith Lynch so aptly described them. A shingled building, No. 636, has pleached ficus street trees in front and around the corner. No. 619, built in 1913, and No. 609, built in 1910, are some of the older homes in this section. A mini park, The Benches, is located at 18th St. You also have a view of Twin Peaks from here. (A skywalk extends across Highway 101.)

- Turn right on 18th St. and left on Vermont. The Slovenian Hall is at the left corner of Vermont at Mariposa. Turn right. The early Greek settlement was in this section. Light industry and small entrepreneurial firms are located in the lowlands north of Mariposa, to your left.

- Continue on Mariposa toward Rhode Island. Turn left on Rhode Island to No. 350, built in 2002 on the site of a recycling center. To give historic perspective, the architect used glass shards as part of the wall in the courtyard. Heavy metal grates hold back the glass. Turn right onto 16th St. A few feet from the corner is the San Francisco Center for the Book. One of the most active chapters in the country, they offer classes in various forms of the book arts, from traditional to experimental; there are classes in the use of the Letter Press, and bookmaking for children is offered. You are welcome to come in to see the exhibits Monday through Friday and attend public events. For more information, call (415) 565-0545.

- Continue on 16th St. to De Haro and turn right. Continue to 500 De Haro, to St. Gregory of Nyssa Episcopal Church built in 1995 and designed by architect John Goldman. St. Gregory parish places strong emphasis on liturgy that is grounded in Jewish and early Christian practice. Their belief in unconditional hospitality, a strong sense of community, and in music and dance, is expressed in the shape of the entrance—a large, octagonal open space, with an encircling mural depicting joyous dancing saints. After the liturgy in the adjoining room, the congregation reenters the open space and dances, reflecting the movements of the saints. A table is set with food for the congregation to partake.

- Across the street at 1705 Mariposa is the home of Anchor Brewing Co., one of the finest small breweries in the country. Its history goes back to the 1860s when it brewed one beer that was available only on tap. Now Anchor produces six handcrafted beers, plus a selection of seasonal beers. Two-hour tours are given Monday through Friday at 1 PM by reservation only. Due to its popularity, four- to six-weeks' notice is generally necessary for a reservation. For more information, call (415) 863-8350.

- Continue on De Haro toward 19th St. You pass Enola D. Maxwell Middle School of the Arts at 655 De Haro, and soon after, an open space that contains remnants of a garden. You can see the Bay Bridge from here.

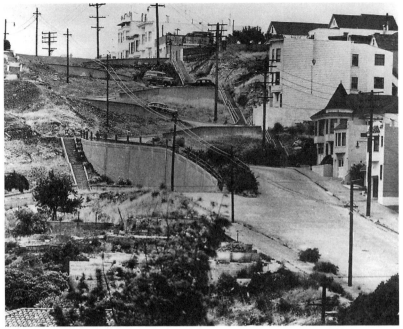

Potrero Hill, ca. 1950 *Courtesy of San Francisco Archives*

- Turn left on 19th St. to Carolina, and then right on Carolina to ascend the Carolina Stairway to 20th St. At the top are redwoods. The right-of-way has evolved into a garden with trees, agave, ivy, and shrubs. The Victoria Mews Association maintains the garden.

- Turn right on 20th St. to De Haro. A large embankment of serpentine rock at the southwest corner is the location of Francisco De Haro's adobe cottage built here in the 1830s. He was chosen as the first Mexican *alcalde* (Spanish for *mayor*) of the Pueblo Yerba Buena in 1834.

- Turn left on De Haro and walk on the left side in order to have a better view of the new architecture on the right.

- Continue on De Haro. Across the street from NABE, a Mini Park is being constructed, where a memorial plaque honors Ruth Davidow, a neighborhood activist. Cross the street to your beginning.

Stairway

Bernal Heights East

Trails

Bernal Heights sits high above a maze of major thoroughfares—Alemany, Mission, and Cesar Chavez streets and Highways 101 and 280. It is part of what was once the Rancho de las Salinas y Potrero Nuevo, granted to Jose Cornelio de Bernal in 1839 by the Mexican government. In the 1860s the rancho (one league square, approximately 4,000 acres) was subdivided and Vitus Wackenreuder made a survey of Bernal Heights. Wackenreuder plotted his streets narrow and his lots small—23 by 76 feet. Most of them do not meet today's City specifications of minimum size. The east slope exceeds a 45% grade in many places, and its geological composition has hazardous landslide potential.

After the area was subdivided, the first settlers were predominantly Irish. They farmed the land and engaged in dairy ranching, the first extensive industry in Bernal Heights. Wakes were the most popular social gatherings, along with the telling of stories by "them as had the gift." The day Widow O'Brien's best milk cow was taken to the city pound and all her neighbors helped her get it back provided a true neighborhood story, endlessly told.

German and Italian settlers followed the Irish. During World War II, there was an influx of people, mainly blue-collar, from all over the United States, who came to work in the nearby naval shipyards. More recently, professionals and media people have been moving into the neighborhood, attracted by the sunny climate and the neighborhood ambiance of the village within the City. Since 1995, the east slope of

Bernal Heights has experienced fundamental and dramatic changes. A capital improvement project from sales tax monies has brought the streets into compliance with mandated safety codes. Along with streets and water lines, the area now has, at this writing, 50-plus stairways, many of them constructed in unused rights-of-way, on hills too steep to construct a street. The east slope is now one grand forest of stairway trails to explore. I encourage you to try out new routes.

The streets of Bernal Heights East meet at angles that vary from the rectangular grid. Also, street names can flip-flop within a block, and several streets converge at a "corner." I have mentioned these facts to several residents, who seem surprised, but they understand the system.

◢ Begin at the "corner" of Peralta 600 and Esmeralda 1000. Across the street is the unmarked Esmeralda Stairway, which you descend to Franconia. New landscaping and new amenities set the tone for an adventure along the improved Bernal Heights stairways. You'll see plum trees and pines, and various annuals. A provided platform enables you to sit on a bench and look toward Hunters Point and the East Bay hills.

◢ Turn right on the 400 block of Franconia. Several redwood-shingled houses dominate the street. Next to No. 447, turn left to the unmarked Mayflower Stairway to Holladay. Two palm trees have been planted at the beginning of the descent. At the next to last landing you have a view of India Basin and Oakland.

◢ Continue down through the driveway to Holladay and turn left. The Bayshore Freeway (Highway 101) traffic noise is mitigated by double-paned windows and other insulation installed in the new and remodeled homes along the street. The slope is privately owned and consists of 13 lots. Some efforts to build were stalled by the neighbors who are hoping to keep it as open space.

◢ Turn left at Joy Stairway, where a corkscrew willow tree has been planted. I have fond memories of the first Joy Stairway—a few steps that led up to a pulpit-like structure, then continued in a haphazard fashion, up to Brewster. The slope was slippery and muddy then because of the heavy rains of 1982–1983. The ambiance was rural, with gingham and calico accents. More than 20 years later, the new pedestrian thoroughfares have been built to conform to safety codes. But No. 18 Joy is an original flat-front Italianate from the 1870s.

▟ Continue up the wood stairway to Brewster. Across from No. 138 Brewster, turn right and descend Faith Stairway. This concrete stairway traverses a garden of sweet peas, poppies, lavender, ceanothus, coast live oaks, and pines. At the top, on the right, No. 159 Faith, built in 1901, features a stained-glass window. No. 137 Faith was connected to water in 1934, and No. 132 Faith in 1944. From here, the skywalk that arches over the Bayshore Freeway looks attractive.

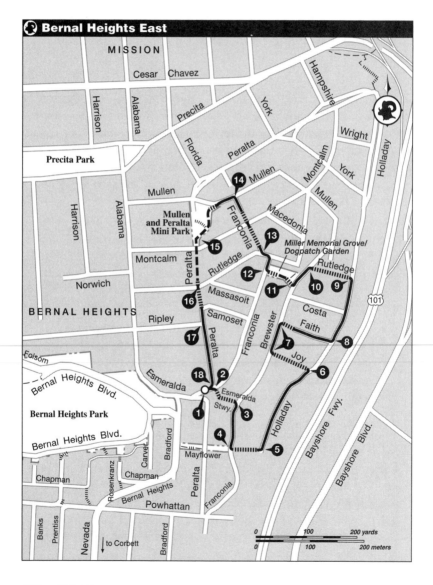

Will Kemp, the Shakespearean clown, jigged the 100 miles from London to Norwich on a bet, in February 1600.

⚐ From the bottom of the stairs continue to Holladay. Turn left on Holladay and walk past Costa to Rutledge Stairway (next to No. 300 Holladay). It is an unmarked street right-of-way. You ascend the timber and metal stairway through a garden of redwoods, pines, a buckeye tree, and annuals. Walk up the concrete stairs. At the top is the cul-de-sac of Mullen.

⚐ To the right, the city land is planted with trees. To the left, the stairway continues where you ascend past some cottages. No. 43 Rutledge, built in 1895, is especially attractive in its setting among garden vines and trees on the lot. No. 55 Rutledge, on the left-side

---

WALK 23 ROUTE: Bernal Heights East

Public Transportation: MUNI Bus #67 Bernal Heights. For MUNI bus information, call 311 (outside San Francisco call (415) 701-2311).

1. Begin at the corner of Peralta 600 and Esmeralda 1000.
2. Veer right to descend the unmarked Esmeralda Stwy.
3. Right on the 400 block of lower Franconia; continue to the right.
4. Left to descend the unmarked Mayflower Stwy.
5. Left on Holladay to Joy Stwy.
6. Left to ascend Joy Stwy. to Brewster.
7. Right on Brewster to Faith Stwy. and descend.
8. Continue to Holladay and turn left.
9. Ascend Rutledge Stwy. next to No. 300 Holladay and continue beyond the Mullen cul-de-sac to Brewster.
10. Left on Brewster to end of the retaining wall.
11. Bear right up the stairway. At first landing, turn left. Ascend stairway through community garden to Franconia.
12. Right on Franconia to Rutledge. Turn left.
13. Descend Franconia Stwy. Cross Montcalm and continue to Mullen.
14. Left on Mullen. Ascend the stairway ramp to the Open Space area. Follow path to Montcalm and Peralta.
15. Cross Montcalm and continue up Peralta walkway. Ascend short stairway to Rutledge.
16. Cross Rutledge to ascend Peralta Stwy.
17. Continue on Peralta past Ripley.
18. Right on Esmeralda to your beginning.

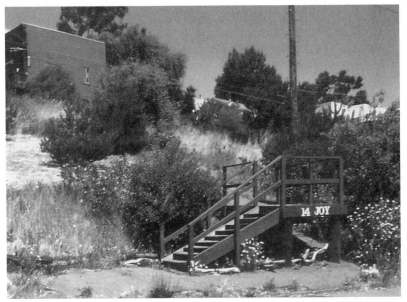

This historical photograph shows the Joy Stairway in 1983. *Adah Bakalinsky*

corner at Brewster, has an old-fashioned porch along the front of the house and some sculptures in the front garden.

◢ Continue left on Brewster and walk past the retaining wall, then turn an immediate right to ascend the stairway. The Miller Memorial Grove/Dogpatch Garden is on your right. You will bear left and ascend the stairway through the Community Garden. At the top, pass through the gate with the sign: THIS IS A NICE NEIGH-BORHOOD GARDEN.

◢ You are now on Franconia. Turn right and then left on Rutledge to descend the stairway to Montcalm. The slope with the newly designed stairway and garden plots is the result of cooperation by neighbors. The project sped along at an amazing rate (one year) due to good planning, excellent collaboration with the Department of Public Works, Division of Street-Use Permits, and some serendipities: One of the neighbors, an architect, facilitated the acquisition of permits by promptly completing the technical drawings required by the City; one of the neighbors is a contractor who donated his employees to build the stairway; and another neighbor assisted with fund-raising and publicity; and San Francisco Beautiful contributed. The ribbon cutting was Sunday, November 14, 2004.

- Cross Montcalm and continue to Mullen. No. 109 Franconia is a Craftsman-style home that has an award-winning garden along Montcalm. Turn left on Mullen. Continue on the left side to ascend the stairway ramp. You pass a Japanese-style compound of several residences, built around a common courtyard.

- Follow the path to the crest of Peralta Point. City street rights-of-way and Open Space funding contributed to this open area's establishment; it provides views of the downtown skyline from the Rincon Tower building to Twin Peaks. Plans are in place for restoring native plants.

- Continue left on the pathway adjacent to the Open Space Garden around the point and walk ahead to Montcalm. Veer right and cross Montcalm. Turn left on Peralta and follow the walkway and short stairway, composed of different-sized and -colored steps.

- Cross Rutledge and ascend the Peralta Stairway. At the top you get a view of San Francisco that always makes me catch my breath. The house on your right has an unusual fan-shaped fence. A redwood tree is at the corner of Samoset and Peralta. Continue on Peralta, past Ripley to Esmeralda and your beginning.

Circling

Bernal Heights West

Two Hills

A sunny neighborhood, Bernal Heights enjoys extraordinary views of the City. With the largest number of stairways of any neighborhood, it also has a greater variety of street names with historic associations than any other. Among them you find: Banks, Winslow, Putnam, Army, Moultrie, and Sumter that relate to the Civil War; Powhattan, Samoset, and Massasoit that relate to Native American leaders; and several that relate to the U.S. Colonial period. Bernal Heights has streets that change names, corners that don't coincide, some unpaved paths, and some of the most dedicated and active neighborhood-watch groups in the City. Neighbors here know how to work and cooperate with City agencies: They have been successful in establishing and preserving open space and community gardens wherever feasible.

- Begin your walk in an unusual circular configuration at Holly Park. Real estate developers gave it to the City in the 1860s hoping that an elite neighborhood would develop here, as it did in South Park, but the neighborhood became working class around 1900.

- Ascend the concrete stairway at Holly Park Circle and Bocana. Follow the circular path clockwise around the park. Rockrose, marguerites, salvia, iris, and boxwood bushes have been planted along the slopes. Holly Hill (274') provides a view around the cardinal points of the compass. Behind you at the Bocana intersection is

Bernal Heights Hill (325'), your destination. You can also see the dark, carnelian granite Bank of America building in the Financial District. Follow the walkway, and at Newman, look for the grove of olive trees transplanted from the Civic Center in 1998 which lines this eastern section of Holly Hill, as does a grove of eucalyptus. Near the Park St. intersection, you see the Bayview District and Hunters Point. Looking south from the Murray intersection you can see the blue water tower in McLaren Park. Continue on the path that dips down to the Appleton intersection, from where you see the buildings of Diamond Heights.

⊿ Cross Holly Park Circle at Appleton, and turn right to Elsie. You pass the College Hill Reservoir, built in the mid-19th century to bring water to the Mission District. Along the sidewalk you also pass Elsie Garden, the work of talented and caring neighbors. At No. 324 Elsie is a jacaranda tree. Turn left at Santa Marina, and turn right next to No. 101 to descend the Prospect Stairway to Cortland. Walk through the Good Prospect Community Garden. It has a great variety of plants: roses, sweet peas, thyme, lemon verbena, Russian sage, vegetables, and fruit trees.

⊿ Continue on Prospect and turn left on Kingston. Follow the walkway to the concrete and steel stairway, built alongside the Franciscan Formation. You can see the nonidentical twin spires of St. Paul's Church in Noe Valley, and above it Diamond Heights and Twin Peaks. Turn right on Coleridge to Eugenia. Walk uphill to the angled Eugenia Stairway, indicated by bollards and a eucalyptus tree, flanked by agave and ivy, and shaded by gingko and pine trees. A sign announces EUGENIA GARDEN.

⊿ At the top you cross Winfield, continue on Eugenia, and turn left at the combination Virginia and Elsie. The street then divides— Virginia goes downhill and Elsie up. Cross the street to No. 199 Elsie. Turn left and walk to the uphill side of the gore point, just past the one-way sign, and cross the street. Walk on the sidewalk to the left of No. 319, the shingled house with tile accents. Follow the Virginia Garden Walk, another neighborhood beautification project.

⊿ Go past the two stairways to your left, follow the left curve, and descend the third stairway. The sign VIRGINIA GARDEN WALK is to the left. Cross Winfield. No. 217 Virginia is a three-story Stick-style Italianate. Continue down mostly elm tree-lined Virginia.

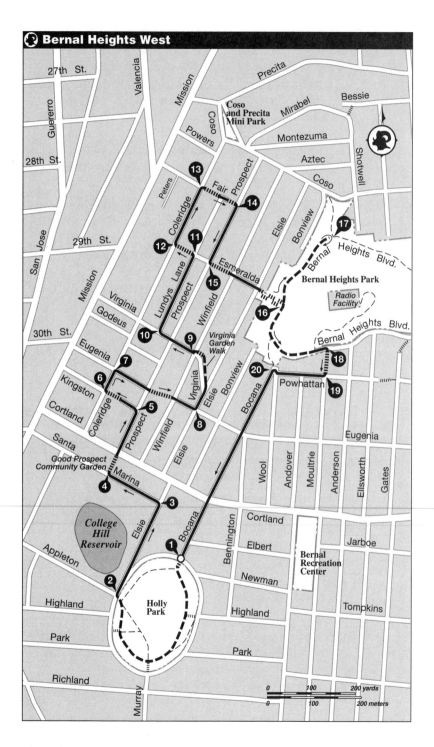

- Pass Prospect and turn right on Lundys Lane, one of my favorite streets. Carob trees planted along the street complement the cottages here.

- Turn left to descend the concrete Esmeralda Stairway, which is enhanced by plantings of ceanothus, sage, and daisies. At the top and bottom of the stairway are viewing platforms.

- Turn right on Coleridge. There is a Mini Park across the street. Continue to Fair; turn right and ascend the Fair Stairway. In 1990, a Cinco de Mayo dance with costumed dancers and live music was performed at the top of the stairway. Continue past the brick-paved cul-de-sac of Lundys Lane.

WALK 24 ROUTE: Bernal Heights West

Public Transportation: MUNI Bus #24 Divisadero. For MUNI bus or Metro information, call 311 (outside San Francisco call (415) 701-2311).

1. Begin at Holly Park Circle and Bocana. Ascend stairway into Holly Park. Walk clockwise on circular path to Appleton and Elsie.
2. Cross Holly Park Circle, turn right and walk to Elsie.
3. Continue on Elsie to Santa Marina. Turn left.
4. Right to descend Prospect Stwy. to Kingston.
5. Left to Kingston Stwy. to Coleridge.
6. Right on Coleridge to Eugenia.
7. Right on Eugenia. At Prospect ascend Eugenia Stwy. to Winfield. Continue to intersection of Virginia and Elsie.
8. Cross the street to No. 199 Elsie. Left to the gore point and cross to No. 319 Virginia.
9. Walk to the end of Virginia Garden Walk. Descend short stairway. Continue past Winfield and Prospect to Lundys Lane.
10. Right on Lundys Lane to Esmeralda.
11. Left to descend Esmeralda Stwy.
12. Right on Coleridge to Fair.
13. Right to ascend Fair Stwy. to Prospect.
14. Right on Prospect to Esmeralda.
15. Left to ascend Esmeralda Stwy. to Bernal Heights Blvd.
16. Left on Bernal Heights Blvd. for views.
17. Return on Bernal Heights Blvd., past Esmeralda, to Moultrie.
18. Right to descend Moultrie Stwy. to Powhattan.
19. Right on Powhattan to Bocana.
20. Left on Bocana to your beginning.

- Turn right on Prospect, next to a garden with pines, eucalyptus, echium, pelargonium, and agapanthus. Continue over the hill past No. 34, one of the oldest homes in Bernal Heights. Situated on the original goat farm, the homestead has been extended from a simple, narrow clapboard with gables to a roomy, two-story, eight-room structure.

- Turn left onto another section of the Esmeralda Stairway—this one with steel handrails and lights, flowers along the edges, and rope swings hanging from the branches of tall trees. At the top of the stairway is the recently refurbished double slide. Adults like to try it, and they quickly arrive at the bottom. Several trees, including a large pepper, shade the picnic table and bench at the Winfield Plaza.

- Continue up the short street block of Esmeralda to the highest section of the stairway.

In 1885 Charles Lummis walked 3,500 miles, from Cincinnati, Ohio, to Los Angeles in 143 days. He paid for his trip by writing articles about his adventures for the Los Angeles Times. *He fought off a wildcat, a mountain lion, escaped from convicts, and set his own broken arm. Subsequently he became city editor of the newspaper.*

- This section of the Esmeralda Stairway leads through a shade garden of ferns and rhododendrons, another project of caring neighbors. A stone monument is marked with a memorial plaque for the late Margaret Randolph, a Bernal Heights activist.

- At the top, surrounded by flowering plum and ceanothus, is the asphalt road that circles Bernal Heights Park. Neighbors succeeded in having the City close this section of road to cars, making it safe for walkers. Designated as a "natural area," the hill is where the Native Plant Society and the Bernal Hilltop Native Grassland Restoration Project have monthly work parties.

- The route around the hill is 1 mile long, and many people jog or walk its length. The view from here is one of the most rewarding in the City. Walk left as far as you like for the views, and then retrace your steps (south) to a west-facing bench where you can take in San Bruno Mountain, Twin Peaks, and Angel Island.

- Walk past Esmeralda and continue on the road as it curves left past the auto barrier. Then walk to the end of the chain-link fence and look for the beginning of the Moultrie Stairway, near the driveway of No. 123 (written on the wood fence), beside the multiple mail-boxes. Bear right at the fence and left under a eucalyptus. The little pebble path with wood water-stop steps becomes a concrete walk that goes past gardens. Walk on a ramp to Powhattan.

- Turn right and proceed along Powhattan to the end. The triangle-shaped garden across the street is a neighbor-initiated project.

- Turn left on Bocana to go downhill toward Holly Park to your beginning. When you cross Cortland, one of the major east-west streets and the major shopping street, you can bear left to an area of coffeehouses and restaurants.

Follow the Curve,

Diamond Heights, Fairmount Heights,

Follow the View

& Glen Canyon Park

The Diamond Heights neighborhood was built on 325 acres of craggy, hilly terrain after World War II, when federal redevelopment money became available for construction. A range of modest-to-luxurious homes, town houses, apartments, and condominiums were built, trees were planted, and stairways were constructed. Diamond Heights is bounded by important corridor streets, O'Shaughnessy, Portola, Clipper, and Diamond Heights Blvd., and by the 300-foot-deep Glen Canyon Park, which separates it from Miraloma to the west and Glen Park to the east.

◢ Beginning at the shopping-center corner of Diamond Heights Blvd. (No. 5290) and Gold Mine, walk right up Diamond Heights Blvd. At the next intersection, turn left on Diamond and follow the curve to Beacon. I love to take visitors here for the remarkable vista. Walk along the ridge of Beacon on the sidewalk until No. 425, then cross the street to a footpath. Here we see cycle tracks and footpaths crisscross the slope of Billy Goat Hill. Bernal Heights Park and its radio tower are seen straight ahead on the hill.

◢ The Harry Stairway begins between Nos. 190 and 200 Beacon. It is very easy to miss because it looks like a private walkway. The stairway is constructed of both wood and concrete. You descend parallel to numerous conifers growing in the lot on the right. Monterey cypress branches overhang the stairway. I like the surprising contrast in atmosphere and vegetation between an urban street and a forest path. The long Harry Stairway lets you see the variety in homes alongside, which establishes an individual style to the vicinity.

- When you're on the lower concrete steps, you will see Yerba Buena Island and the Bay Bridge to the east, and the spires of St. Paul's Church and downtown San Francisco north. All the while, nearest you, African daisies, ivy, geraniums, wild onion, pittisporum, yucca, lily of the Nile, datura, abutilon, nasturtium, and hydrangeas provide a celebration of color and foliage.

- The Harry Stairway ends at Laidley No. 100. You are now in the Fairmount Heights neighborhood that was platted in 1864. The boundaries are Castro to the west, Arlington to the east, 30th to the north, and Bemis to the south. Cobb and Sinton were the real estate developers. Old photos show vernacular cottages along unpaved paths and pine groves.

Harry Stairway *Tony Holiday*

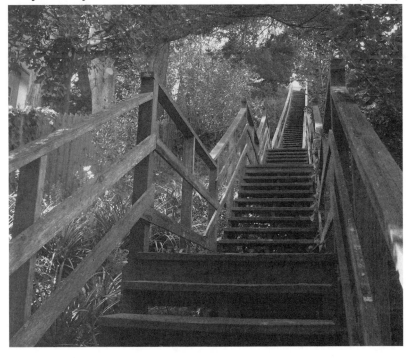

Diamond Heights, Fairmount Heights, & Glen Canyon Park **189**

■ Turn right on Laidley. A short street (one of my favorites), it is, essentially, a street of cottages. A resident of the street, architect Jeremy Kotas has been responsible for the dramatic metamorphosis from simple cottages to imaginative, contemporary dwellings. You pass several homes he worked on: Nos. 102, 128, 134, 123, 140, and 135.

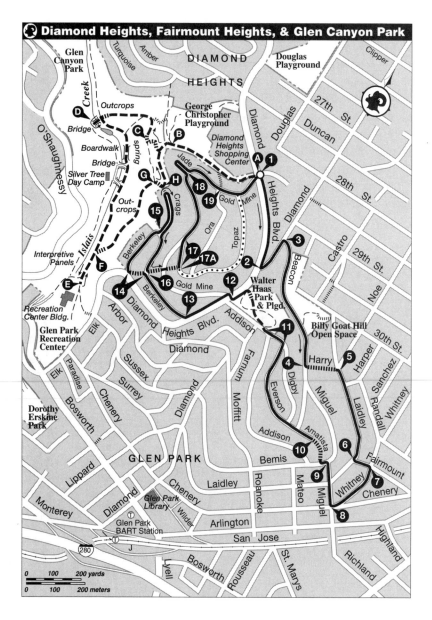

WALK 25 ROUTE: Diamond Heights, Fairmount Heights, & Glen Canyon Park

Public Transportation: MUNI Bus #35 Eureka; #52 Excelsior. The Glen Park BART station is in the area. For MUNI bus information, call 311 (outside San Francisco call (415) 701-2311).

1. From Diamond Heights Blvd. shopping center (No. 5290) and Gold Mine, walk south on Diamond Heights Blvd. to Diamond St.

2. Left on Diamond St. to Beacon.

3. Right on Beacon to Harry Stwy., next to No. 190 Beacon.

4. Descend stairway to Laidley.

5. Right on Laidley.

6. Left on Fairmount.

7. Right on Whitney.

8. Right to Chenery, and right again on Miguel.

9. Left on Bemis, and then right to ascend Amatista Stwy. to Everson.

10. Bear left on Everson. Continue to end of street at DIGBY 000 sign.

11. Turn left on Digby, cross Addison. Right into Haas Park and left to ascend stairway to Diamond Heights Blvd.

12. Cross the Blvd. Left on Diamond Heights Blvd. to Berkeley Way.

13. Right on Berkeley Way.

14. Next to No. 101, left to descend Onique Stwy. Right on Berkeley Way and cross street to see canyon and rock formation near corner of Crags Ct. Bear right.

15. Turn left. Go to end of Crags Ct. Return to Berkeley Way. Bear left.

16. Next to No. 100 Berkeley Way, ascend Onique Stwy. (left) to No. 400 Gold Mine. Continue up Onique Stwy. to No. 243 Topaz.

17. Left on Topaz. Right on Gold Mine.

17A. *Optional:* Right on Topaz. Right on Gold Mine to your beginning.

18. Walk into Jade Place and return to Gold Mine.

19. Continue on Gold Mine to Diamond Heights Blvd. to your beginning.

A. Walk in area from Diamond Heights Blvd. and Gold Mine Drive to George Christopher Playground along the path to the left.

B. Take the left path into the canyon and descend first log and plank stairway.

C. Continue on paths and log and plank stairways toward the right. The path will end on the road near the bridge.

D. Left to cross bridge and boardwalk. Continue walking on either side of Islais Creek toward the Glen Park Recreation Center building.

E. The interpretive panel near the recreation center outlines the trails in the canyon: Christopher Park, Crags Court, and Berkeley Way.

F. To return, walk to the next interpretive panel by the light post. Ascend path with log and plank stairways, continuing along the outcrops toward Crags Court.

G. Continue on right path at junction and ascend toward Crags Court.

H. Just before Crags Court, turn left on path back to your beginning.

No. 134 is the Sand Castle because of the undulating first story, and No. 140 is known in the neighborhood as the Owl House because of the curving features that resemble eyebrows.

A walk should have simplicity and complexity,
contrast and unity.

—A. Packerman

◢ The palatial three-story, Second Empire and Italianate home, Nos. 192–196 (near Fairmount), now an apartment house, was built in 1872. It is commonly known as the Bell Mystery House. The death of the owner, Thomas Bell, a San Francisco financier, occurred under mysterious circumstances in 1892. His wife, Teresa, and his housekeeper, Mary Ann Pleasant, may have been involved. Without a satisfactory explanation, it has been fodder for a neighborhood myth. Pleasant (known as Mammy Pleasant) is the most interesting character in the story. A free-born black woman from Philadelphia, dedicated abolitionist, and entrepreneur, she was a celebrated cook who worked for wealthy families. She owned laundries, boardinghouses, and brothels. (For more information about her, see *Mammy Pleasant* and *Mammy Pleasant's Partner* both by Helen Holdredge and *A Cast of Hawks* by Milton Gould.)

◢ Turn left on Fairmount. No. 226 is a "tuck-in," set deep into the lot where residents can enjoy an enviable view. Make a right turn on Whitney, a small street with several row Queen Annes. Turn right to Chenery, the Glen Park neighborhood shopping street. Farther along the street, a coffeehouse, a bakery, the hardware store, and Bird & Beckett Books and Records convey the essence of a small town Main Street. A new branch library was opened in February 2010 at 2825 Diamond.

◢ Turn right on Miguel and walk uphill to Bemis. Turn left and then right to ascend the Amatista Stairway to Everson. A shopping center was proposed for the triangle near the top of the stairs, but residents opposed it, and the area is now a small park.

◢ Everson is one of the oldest sections of the Diamond Heights Redevelopment Area. A resident told me that her home and the house at No. 50 Everson, which was made with lumber from the 1939 Golden Gate International Exposition on Treasure Island, were the only two structures on the street in 1957.

- Continue on the left side of Everson for the view: Bayview Heights, the blue water tower of the Excelsior neighborhood, and San Bruno Mountain with its radio towers. Walk past the DIGBY 100 street sign. Continue to the end of Everson at the DIGBY 000 sign.

- Turn left, pass the fire station, cross Addison, and walk right through the basketball court of the four-plus-acre Walter Haas Park and Playground, an inviting place for picnicking, playing, and just sitting.

- Walk up the short stairway to Diamond Heights Blvd. If you'd like to return to the beginning of the walk at this point, turn right. If you'd like to continue on the Diamond Heights portion of the walk, cross the boulevard and turn left. You pass a sign that reads GOLD MINE 000 END. Continue on Diamond Heights Blvd. to Berkeley Way.

- At Berkeley Way turn right. Next to No. 101, descend Onique Stairway to the lower loop of Berkeley Way. Turn right on Berkeley Way and cross the street. You are looking down on Glen Canyon Park, where, in the 1800s, carnivals, parades, picnics, dances, and other amusements took place. Continue farther to see the extraordinary rock formation near the corner of Crags Court. One of the first residents on Crags bought a house here to practice rock climbing.

- Veer right and turn left at the corner. Continue to the end of Crags. A thriving community garden exists in this area now. The people who attend it welcome visitors and will share their knowledge and samples of fruits and flowers.

To Crags Court *Tony Holiday*

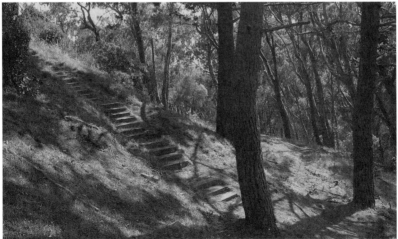

Diamond Heights, Fairmount Heights, & Glen Canyon Park **193**

- Return to the upper loop of Berkeley Way. Eucalyptus and pine trees have been planted here and in the hills (right) above O'Shaughnessy. Walk on the left side. Next to No. 100 Berkeley Way, ascend Onique Stairway. Midway you're next to No. 400 Gold Mine. Cross the street and continue upward. At the top we are next to No. 243 Topaz.

- Turn left on Topaz and right on Gold Mine (679'). Turn left into Jade Place for mini-views of the Sutro Tower, Mt. Davidson, and San Bruno Mountain between the houses and garages. As you return to Gold Mine you are confronted by the incongruous placement of the Rincon Towers next to our iconic Bay Bridge, my Cinderella bridge. It's a carrier of heavy traffic during the day and, in the evening, a graceful structure within the bridge lights. Continue around to your left, walking downhill on Gold Mine to the beginning.

- An optional route, which I like very much, is to turn right on Topaz. As you walk along the ridge near No. 131, an extraordinary view unfolds before you—east and south. Continue down the hill to Gold Mine; bear right to your beginning.

- You may want to take the alternate route in Glen Canyon Park (Steps A–H on the map) upon your return to Diamond Heights Blvd., or perhaps you prefer to enjoy it at another time. Watch your step because the paths are narrow. You may want to use a walking stick.

- During periods of heavy rain or restoration work in Glen Canyon, you cannot walk along the left side of Islais Creek. However, by walking on the main road (the right side), you can see the plants that grow so well near and in water—willows, sedges, and equisetum. You can see the native wildflowers growing on the slopes of the hill—sticky monkeyflower, coyote brush, red flowering currant, and columbine. By walking across the wood bridge, you can see the many birds, the walkers, and their dogs and enjoy at close range the 300-foot canyon in the middle of the City, which exposes the massive Franciscan Formation.

Further Ambling

Chenery, the "downtown" Glen Park, has the atmosphere of a small town main street. There are restaurants and stores. Visit the new library at 2825 Diamond at Wilder.

A Harmonious

McLaren Park & Excelsior

Walk

McLaren Park, located in the southeast corner
of San Francisco, is the City's second largest park
(318 acres) and one of its least known. In this walk
you'll explore the seeps, ponds, and marshes of the
park's well-tended northern edge. By traversing bridges
and stairways you'll segue into the surrounding neighborhood, which still retains a relatively rustic ambiance. All these
elements mingle harmoniously here.

The park was dedicated to John McLaren, who was the chief gardener of Golden Gate Park for 60 years. While land purchases for the
park began in the late 1920s, its designated area was not fully acquired
until the 1970s, due to short funding and dozens of farming inhold-
ings. In 1987 a bond issue providing $2.4 million to implement the
master plan for McLaren Park was passed. It provided for a felicitous
park design, with cypress and redwood groves, cattail marshes, and
riparian areas where willow and horsetail grow.

⬛ Begin in the 300 block of Gambier at Felton and walk toward
Burrows. The attached houses on your left date from the 1940s and
1950s, but on the right are cottages of the early 1900s. They occupy
two or three lots with room for extensive yards and outbuildings.
Gravel driveways and well-tended gardens lend them a rural
touch.

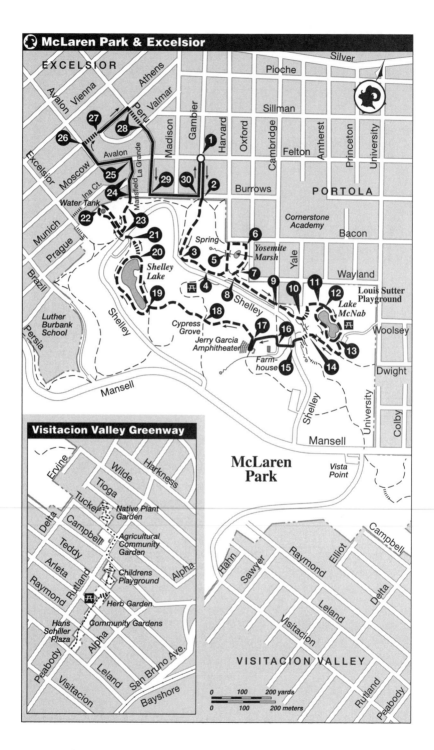

WALK 26 ROUTE: McLaren Park & Excelsior

Public Transportation: MUNI Bus #52 Excelsior, #54 Felton. For MUNI bus information, call 311 (outside San Francisco call (415) 701-2311).

1. Begin in 300 block of Gambier at Felton. Walk to Burrows.
2. Cross Burrows into McLaren Park. Continue straight on descending path.
3. Follow curve of trail along a eucalyptus grove and then a redwood grove.
4. Continue left from sandbox.
5. Cross a concrete bridge.
6. Continue around left edge of Yosemite Marsh on asphalt path.
7. Right at basketball court.
8. Left to go along path beside Shelley.
9. Cross Cambridge and continue on path; bear left at next junction.
10. Descend stairway to Yale.
11. Right and descend driveway to Lake McNab.
12. Walk either way around Lake McNab.
13. Leave lake via sandy playground in Louis Sutter Playground. Bear right on paved path.
14. After the footbridge, take left path and railroad-tie stairway; then bear right on side path to Shelley.
15. Cross Shelley and walk up paved driveway opposite.
16. Right, then left to parking lot and view amphitheater.
17. Return to parking lot gate. Bear left to go up the gravel path.
18. At path and trail intersection, bear left on gravel path; continue ahead at the cypress grove junction on the level path.
19. At south tip of Shelley Lake, walk either way around the lake.
20. At north end turn left. Climb long railroad-tie stairway to crest of the hill.
21. Continue past parking lot to Shelley; cross it and ascend long paved driveway.
22. Circle counterclockwise around water tower.
23. Retrace steps to Shelley. Turn left on paved path. Stay left at playground.
24. Exit park at corner of Burrows and Mansfield. Continue straight on Mansfield, which turns into La Grande, for one block.
25. Left on Avalon. Continue on Avalon one block to Moscow, and right for one block more to Athens.
26. Right; ascend Athens Stwy.
27. Continue on Athens for one block to Peru.
28. Ascend Peru Stwy. to Valmar. Continue on Peru for two blocks to Burrows.
29. Left on Burrows to Gambier.
30. Left to 300 block of Gambier to your beginning.

*"I love walking in London," said Mrs. Dalloway. "Really it's
better than walking in the country."*
　　　　　　　　—from *Mrs. Dalloway* by Virginia Woolf

- Enter McLaren Park from Burrows and Gambier. A neighbor enjoying the view from his porch told me the park across the street was rough pasture when he moved here in 1961; he still feels as if he lives in the country.

- Proceed straight on an asphalt walkway that soon begins to descend around the top of a large grassy bowl. Along the trail are eucalyptus and Monterey pine groves (remnants of farm-era wood lots). Follow the curve of the trail along the redwood grove and by young live oak. Keep left along the path parallel to Shelley. You glimpse the Portola and Bayview neighborhoods and the East Bay hills.

- Where the path meets wide Shelley Drive, there's a round sandbox in the middle. Across the street (right) is a large, group picnic area. Proceed left from the sandbox, keeping left along the path.

- The path enters a grove of alder and redwood and crosses a concrete bridge. The creek below flows from a natural spring, just ahead to your left. Look for the horsetails (equisetum). To see where it flows, turn right at the corner of Harvard and Bacon, walk for one block, and turn right again. On your right is a tiny pond filled with cattails. The water's surface is nearly covered with a floating carpet of duckweed. Though human-made, the pond is home to raccoons and small birds. It captures runoff from the grassy bowl you descended from Gambier and keeps the adjacent neighborhood dry.

- Continue around the left edge of the Yosemite Marsh on the asphalt path. Picnic tables, benches, a walkway, and plantings along the pond are some of the inviting aspects of this section. Beyond the round restroom, turn right at the basketball court and clamber up a steep path to some large cypress trees.

- Now turn left and saunter along the path beside Shelley Drive, enjoying the broad views. Behind you is the pond; to your left is the Portola District. The tall, Italian-style tower is Cornerstone Academy, a private school occupying a former convent. To the east you can see the flat expanse of the University Mound Reservoir and get a glimpse of San Francisco Bay and the East Bay hills.

At the intersection of Shelley and Cambridge, cross Cambridge and descend a winding asphalt path through a dense pine grove. Bear left at the next two junctions. Railroad-tie steps descend to the end of Yale. Turn right and descend the paved driveway to Lake McNab, a human-made lake fed by natural springs and runoff from the north slope of McLaren Park. Two big cattail "islands" provide cover for many kinds of birds, including egrets, herons, ducks, and coots. Neighbors enjoy the stroll around the paved lakeshore. The California Conservation Corps is working on two new islands for bird nesting and habitat in this area.

Walk either way around the lake to the far end, where you find a wood-topped drain cover, as well as some swings and a small sandbox in the Louis Sutter Playground; picnic tables provide a pleasant place to sit. Leaving the lake via the sandbox playground, you ascend (right) on a paved path leading past a thicket of willow and alder. Just beyond the first zigzag footbridge, take the left path with railroad-tie steps. Bear right on the short side path to wide Shelley Drive.

Cross Shelley carefully and walk up the paved driveway opposite the Jerry Garcia Amphitheater. About 100 feet up the driveway take the right fork. Turn left at the first opening and follow the parking sign through the small lot for the handicapped. Ahead (left) is the stunning, renovated amphitheater. The Friends of the Jerry Garcia Amphitheater are working to increase the number and types of events held there. Past performances have featured the Bitches Brew, Melvin Seals and the JGB, and Loco Bloco.

After viewing the amphitheater, return to the parking lot gate and follow the gravel path to the left. As you climb, the path goes left through open grassland. Red-tailed hawks sometimes perch on the trees on the right of the path. At a cypress grove near the top of the hill is a complex intersection of paths and trails. Continue straight ahead on the level path crossing a grassy slope edged with coyote brush. In the spring, native wildflowers are abundant (look but don't pick!). Below (right) is the group picnic area you saw near the beginning of the walk.

Your path leads to the south tip of Shelley Lake, a reservoir for the park's irrigation water. This lake is windier and more exposed than other sections of the park. A chain-link fence incompletely separates the lake (several openings let you get close to the water) from the rocky shoreline. Walk along either shore. At the north end, turn left and climb a long railroad-tie stairway to the crest of the hill.

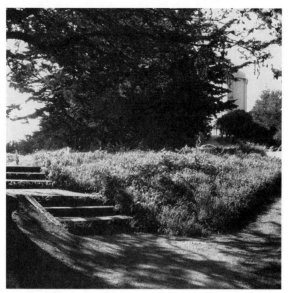

Shelly Lake Stairway *Adah Bakalinsky*

Continue past the parking lot to Shelley. The blue Excelsior water tower, a 50-year-old neighborhood landmark is on the hilltop ahead. The new tank was installed in 2007 and has the same water capacity—350,000 gallons. The water is from Hetch Hetchy Reservoir in the Sierra and is for San Francisco's drinking water and fire protection. Cross Shelley and ascend the long paved driveway. Circle counterclockwise around the water tower to enjoy the panoramic view, one of the grandest in the City. To the north are Bernal Heights, Diamond Heights, Glen Canyon, and Twin Peaks, plus a bit of downtown skyline. To the west is City College, and to the south is the Excelsior District and San Bruno Mountain.

When you are ready, retrace your steps toward Shelley and turn left on the paved path. Stay left at the playground and exit the park at the corner of Burrows and Mansfield. Take a look at No. 73 Mansfield, an unassuming little country house.

Walk ahead one block on Mansfield, and then bear right on La Grande to Avalon. The church on the corner was formerly a neighborhood grocery store. Turn left on Avalon and follow it (as it curves right) to Athens. Turn right and ascend the concrete Athens Stairway. City College gradually comes into view. Continue on Athens for one block to Peru. Your view ahead is toward the northeast.

◢ Ascend Peru Stairway. The adjoining hillside was a dumping ground and an eyesore in the 1970s until a grassroots group, the Hilltop Block Club, banded together. In cooperation with the Recreation and Park Department and the City's Open Space committee, the club retained landscape architect Richard Schadt to design the hillside garden and stairway. Approximately 70 neighborhood residents cooperated in digging, planting, and watering more than 150 trees and shrubs, which had been propagated at the Golden Gate Park nursery. The basic work was completed in 1982.

◢ The serpentine stairway is built of aggregate and railroad ties. The trees on the slopes include Australian willow (*Myoporum*), Italian pine, and flowering plum. The view behind you includes Mt. Davidson (with the cross, Walk 13) and Glen Canyon Park (Walk 25).

◢ You enter an open grassy knoll at the top, Valmar Terrace (a perfect place to sit and read or simply gaze around). The neighbor on the left tends the area, watering, picking up garbage, and planting flowers on her adjoining lot so everyone can enjoy the greenery.

◢ Continue on Peru. (The view now takes in San Francisco General Hospital, the shipyards, Mt. Diablo across the Bay and, to the left, Roundtop Peak.) No. 747 Peru is below street level. Lemon trees grow in the yard, and a penthouse faces east. To the right you see the blue water tower in McLaren Park again, and as you continue walking on Peru, you face the park.

◢ At Peru and Burrows the uneven macadam and adjoining McLaren Park can make you feel like you've been out for a country walk. Turn left on Burrows to reach Gambier to your beginning.

Further Ambling

Visitacion Valley Greenway is one of the finest examples of community work in San Francisco of neighborhood beautification, gardens, and parks that I know. It is difficult not to return time after time to this two-acre greenway developed from six publicly owned lots and extending over a six-block area. Each block has a specialized garden, sculptures, benches, and tiles. The project has taken 16 years. The first five years were spent aquiring properties from the Public Utilities Commission. The next 11 years were spent building the structures and landscaping. In 2009 the last garden, an herb garden, was opened. Fran Martin and Anne Seeman were the prime movers. The decorative

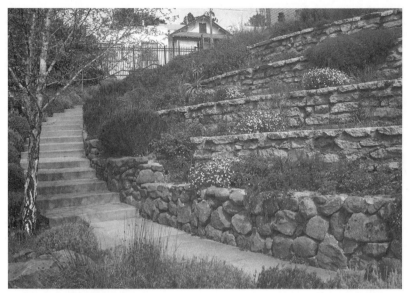

Visitacion Valley Greenway *Annette Hovie*

gates, fences, and tile work were done by sculptor Jim Growden and Fran.

The gardens begin on Leland Ave. across from Peabody St. at Hans Schiller Plaza in the business district. Then they wind through the neighborhood from Raymond to Tioga between Alpha and Delta from Community Garden to Herb Garden to Children's Play Garden to Agricultural Garden to Native Plant Garden.

Views, Views, Views!

Four Hills

A Hop from Hill to Hill

I am convinced that a good walk takes on the shape of *something* real. When I first started working with walking maps, I discovered that the walks I most enjoyed evolved into the shape of a boot or a shoe. My friend Charles Brock who designed the current walk found something else—the Rabbit Hop. It encircles the Upper Market and the Twin Peaks areas. Don't forget to bring your binoculars. It's easy to forget that San Francisco has views all around its perimeter, not just from Telegraph Hill, Russian Hill, and Twin Peaks. To walk in San Francisco is an adventure.

If you want additional information about the neighborhoods, as well many of the streets and highlights, on the Four Hills route, refer to the following four walks: Walk 20: Eureka Valley for Kite Hill; Walk 17: Twin Peaks Foothills for Tank Hill; Walk 18: Upper Market for Mt. Olympus; and Walk 19: Corona Heights for the Corona Heights Hill. For those sections not covered in detail elsewhere in the book, enjoy discovering what catches your eye as you experience the walk.

To walk alone in London is the greatest rest.
—from *The Diary of Virginia Woolf*

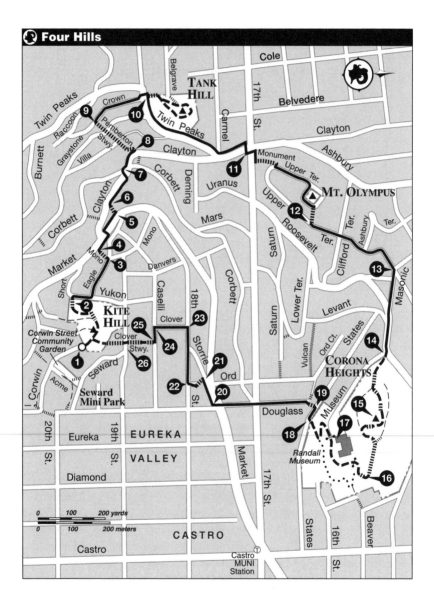

WALK 27 ROUTE: Four Hills

Public Transportation: MUNI Bus #37 Corbett. For MUNI bus information, call 311 (outside San Francisco call (415) 701-2311).

1. Start at the end of Corwin adjacent to Kite Hill Open Space. Enter park and follow trail around to the left and descend stairway and trail to Yukon.
2. Right on Yukon, and immediate left on Eagle.
3. Opposite No. 84 Eagle, ascend Mono Stwy. to Market.
4. Right on Market to Clayton arterial stop. Cross Market at crosswalk.
5. Right down Market 250 feet, then left and ascend stairway to Clayton.
6. Right on Clayton to Corbett.
7. Cross Clayton, then Corbett, and walk up Clayton on the left side.
8. Look left and ascend the Pemberton Stwy. to Crown Terrace.
9. Right on Crown Terrace to Twin Peaks Blvd.
10. Cross Twin Peaks Blvd. at crosswalk and ascend stairway to Tank Hill. Return to Twin Peaks Blvd. and go left to 17th St. and Clayton.
11. Right on 17th St., then immediate left to ascend Monument Way Stwy. Bear left, then right around Mt. Olympus.
12. Next to No. 480 descend stairway to Upper Terrace and turn left to Masonic.
13. Right on Masonic, then straight ahead to Roosevelt and Museum Way.
14. Enter gate in fence. Stay right across lawn and ascend stairways and trail to the summit of Corona Heights.
15. Continue down from summit on stairway, then left on trail, and then right to descend long stairway to trail junction above tennis courts.
16. Head straight for the back porch of the Randall Museum. Cross over the porch and around the museum to the parking lot. Museum is closed Sunday and Monday.
17. Bear left and descend an asphalt path to States.
18. Right on States to No. 187, then left to descend stairway to Douglass.
19. Walk down Douglass and cross Market at crosswalk.
20. Right on Market to Storrie.
21. Left to descend stairway to Ord and 18th St.
22. Right on 18th St. to Clover.
23. Left on Clover to Caselli.
24. Left on Caselli to No. 101.
25. Right to ascend Clover Lane Stwy. and alley to 19th St.
26. Cross 19th St. and ascend narrow stairway and steep trail in Kite Hill Open Space to your beginning.

Jazz

Sunnyside

& Beyond

Some walks feel bouncy, some feel fettered and bound, and others feel as though they will never end. The best walks have a lilt to them. I always try to design walks that have a rhythm, a feeling for the terrain, for the foliage, the rocks, and the rooftops.

Musicians throughout the ages have composed music relating to their environment. Beethoven did that beautifully in his *Sixth Symphony*, Vivaldi in *The Four Seasons*, Art Tatum and his *Lullaby of the Leaves*, Herbie Mann's *A Dance at the Rise of the Moon*, and Bobby Hutcherson's *Highway 1*. Children make up songs about their environment through their everyday activities—jumping rope, shooting marbles, and picking blackberries along the hillside. Adults hum songs describing the physical work they are engaged in. The work songs of slaves are examples of the need for music to give a rhythm to ease physical and mental strain. So it seems natural to me, that while walking, I think and move to the music of the walk. I thought it would be fun to walk a jazz walk. I can't compose a jazz piece, but I can combine some favorite pieces into a coherent selection.

Sunnyside neighborhood is wedged between Balboa Park and Glen Canyon Park. The homes are small, but well taken care of, and all of the front yards are stunning with succulents of varied colors and concentric designs. No. 12 Baden is an earthquake shack from 1907. No. 163 Mangels and No. 330 Congo date to 1899. No. 257 Joost was built in 1900. This jazz route has the contrast that can translate into music.

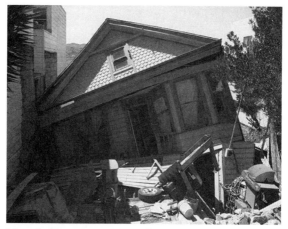

Mangled house on Mangels   *Peter Wanger*

◢ We begin our walk at Mangels and Nordhoff, next to a vacant lot. Four years ago when a group of us were exploring the neighborhood, we saw the house in the lot leaning heavily into the next house. Neighbors were gathered in groups around the house, plus trucks and workmen. Three hours later when we walked back to check on it, there was no house here. The new owner had bought it at a court auction with the warnings, "as is" and "enter at your own risk," and when he was working on the foundation, it gave way, crashing into the house next to it. The poignancy of the pain and distress of the event permeates the walk for me. I keep hearing the saxophone and trumpet wails in Terence Blanchard's *A Tale of God's Will* (A requiem for Katrina).

◢ Next to the lot, on the right, a sign, JOOST & BADEN MINI PARK STAIR-WAY, leads us to a short descent into a garden of succulents, asters, geraniums, sages of different colors, and shrubs and trees, a fairyland park. It is a surprise. Curving corners and greenery edging the curbstones give an additional sense of privacy and of comfort. Continue walking through the levels of the garden to Joost. This seems the perfect place for the sparkling piano of Art Tatum playing *Humoresque.*

◢ At the Joost Mini Park sign, turn left and walk a few yards to the iron gate between Nos. 233 and 241 Joost. Descend the stairway into the Sunnyside Conservatory Park. The Sunnyside Conservatory is a two-story octagonal structure dating from the 1890s. It was built on a subdivided dairy farm lot. When the

Van Beck family bought the property in 1919, it is reported that the area around it was covered with foliage; they discovered the Conservatory only by looking for their lost dog who was trapped inside!

◢ Interest in the Conservatory was ignited in 1973 when new owners applied for a permit to demolish the building. The Sunnyside Neighborhood Association was organized, and the building was given Landmark Status No. 78. Finally after many mishaps (you can read about the history posted on the building wall to the right), the Friends of Sunnyside Conservatory was formed in 1999. They sponsored workdays, art classes, and community events. The City, impressed by the excellent plans of the Friends, the Park and Rec, and the gigantic efforts of many volunteers, awarded 4 million dollars in 2006 for renovation work. On December 5, 2009, the Grand Reopening of the Sunnyside Conservatory took place. The two-story high-ceilinged center octagon basks in natural light from the windows surrounding it on all sides. This large interior room, ordinarily locked, is available for rental and special functions.

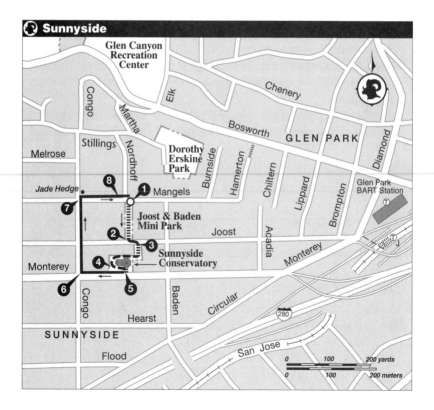

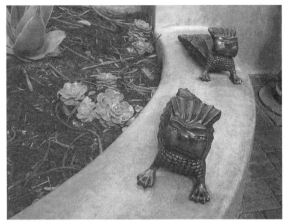

Menagerie Project *Tony Holiday*

◢ Continue around the structure where a variety of succulents and ferns, mallows, geraniums, African lilies, and impatiens have been planted. A magnolia tree and the heritage palms, Canary Island, Chilean Wine, and Norfolk Island, enrich the experience of the Conservatory Park tour.

◢ A special feature of the park is the Menagerie Project designed by Scott Constable and Ene Osteraas-Constable of Wowhaus, a well-known and celebrated art and sculpture team. A doorknob in the shape of a squirrel, and other fanciful creatures are at their ease around the grounds among the plants and embedded in the concrete. The Friends feel the revival of the Conservatory Park far

WALK 28 ROUTE: Sunnyside

Public Transportation: MUNI Bus #23 Monterey, #36 Teresita. For MUNI bus information, call 311 (outside San Francisco call (415) 701-2311).

1. Begin at Mangels across from Nordhoff. Descend stairway into Joost & Baden Mini Park to Joost.
2. Cross Joost. Continue left for a few yards.
3. Enter arched gate to Sunnyside Conservatory Park, between Nos. 233 and 241 Joost. Descend groups of stairways to the Conservatory.
4. Walk around conservatory building. Descend stairway to Monterey Blvd.
5. Right to Congo.
6. Right and continue up the hill to Mangels.
7. Cross street at Mangels to the jade hedge.
8. Continue to Baden to your beginning.

exceeds their expectations. I've seen the area when it was at its lowest point of disrepair. I could not imagine it in its present state of splendor. The setting and the building are perfect for the Haydn *Piano Sonata in F Major* played by Vladimir Horowitz.

◢ Descend the stairway to Monterey Blvd. Turn right on Monterey and continue to Congo. There is a fine view of San Bruno Mountain and the radio towers at the corner and as you walk up the right side of Congo to Joost. Continue to Mangels and cross the street to the jade hedge on the corner. The hedge, full of blooms, is a perfect example of the right plant, right weather, and right growing conditions. At the corner breaking through the wood fence is a deformed tree. As you walk toward Baden, a multicolored stone wall and terraced garden come into view. Continue to your beginning.

Past, Present,

THE BLUE GREENWAY

& Future

Although this book focuses on neighborhood walks in the hill sections of San Francisco, I thought I would like to try a flat walk. The newly developing Mission Bay neighborhood in the southeast section of San Francisco interests me. It includes residences and businesses, a University of California campus, Mission Creek, and the Blue Greenway. A community has begun.

The Blue Greenway is a planned waterfront trail along the Bay shoreline that will complete San Francisco's portion of the Bay Trail. It will connect existing green spaces with new ones and link land and water resources for the enjoyment of nature and recreation. The exciting aspect of the Blue Greenway is that it is progressing toward fulfillment.

Corinne Woods, resident of the Mission Creek neighborhood, has lived in her floating home since 1987. She became an activist for Mission Bay and the Port's waterfront planning. When the Mission Bay Park system is complete, approximately 49 acres of open space will be available for use by the general public.

In 1996 Isabel Wade organized the Neighborhood Parks Alliance, the City's foremost park advocacy group. In 2005, the group launched the Blue Greenway Initiative and the mayor created a task force. Corinne teamed up with Isabel, and has been working as chief advocate for the Blue Greenway. When Corinne walked us through her route, I knew it was the result of many years of exploring.

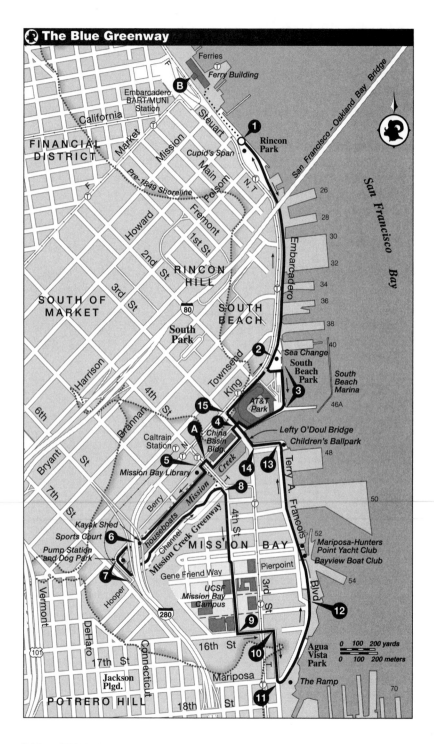

The Blue Greenway

Ferries
Ferry Building

Embarcadero BART/MUNI Station

California

FINANCIAL DISTRICT

Market

Mission

Howard

Folsom

Pre-1849 Shoreline

Cupid's Span

Rincon Park

San Francisco – Oakland Bay Bridge

San Francisco Bay

N. T

Main

Fremont

1st St

2nd St

3rd St

RINCON HILL

80

SOUTH OF MARKET

Embarcadero

SOUTH BEACH

South Park

26
28
30
32
34
36
38
40

Harrison

6th

4th St

Townsend

King

South Beach Park

Sea Change

AT&T Park

South Beach Marina

46A

Brannan St

Bryant St

7th St

Caltrain Station

China Basin Bldg.

Mission Bay Library

Creek

Lefty O'Doul Bridge

Children's Ballpark

48

Terry A. Francois

Berry

houseboats

Channel

Mission

Mission Creek Greenway

MISSION BAY

4th St

50

Kayak Shed
Sports Court

Pump Station and Dog Park

Hooper

Gene Friend Way

Pierpoint

3rd St

52

Mariposa-Hunters Point Yacht Club

Bayview Boat Club

54

Vermont

DeHaro

Connecticut

280

UCSF Mission Bay Campus

Blvd.

12

17th St

Jackson Plgd.

16th St

Mariposa

Agua Vista Park

The Ramp

0   100   200 yards
0   100   200 meters

POTRERO HILL

18th St

70

1
B
2
3
15
A
4
5
14
13
8
6
7
9
10
11

◢ We begin our walk at Rincon Park on the Embarcadero between Howard and Folsom. What a greeting! *Cupid's Span*, the audacious, unconventional sculpture of Claes Oldenburg and Coosje van Bruggen placed in the center of the park for all to see and react to. I wanted to dance around it. The park was developed by Gap, Inc.; the sculpture was commissioned by Donald and Doris Fisher, the company's founders.

◢ Walk along the Embarcadero past Red's Java House at Pier 30. It opened in 1923 as a lunchroom for longshoremen and waterfront

---

WALK 29 ROUTE: The Blue Greenway

Public Transportation: MUNI Metro T Line; F Embarcadero; N Judah; Bus #1 California. If ending at King Street, your bus options include: Townsend and 3rd St. #10 Townsend, Townsend and 4th St. near the Caltrain Station (Muni Bus #30 Stockton, #45 Union, #47 Van Ness, T Line), and King at 4th St. (Muni Bus N Line weekdays only). For MUNI bus or metro information, call 311 (outside San Francisco call (415) 701-2311).

Parking: Minimal and expensive. I recommend public transportation.

1. Begin at Rincon Park on the Embarcadero between Howard and Folsom at the *Cupid's Span* sculpture. Walk along the Embarcadero to Pier 40.
2. Continue to 2nd St. and Townsend to the *Sea Change* sculpture. Walk around South Beach Park, South Beach Harbor, and South Beach Yacht Club.
3. Walk around South Beach Marina to the back of AT&T Park to 3rd St. at Lefty O'Doul Bridge.
4. Cross 3rd St. at crosswalk. Continue on promenade along Mission Creek to 4th St.
5. Cross 4th St. at crosswalk. Continue on Mission Creek past the floating homes.
6. Walk to the path by the kayak storage building. Continue around the sports fields.
7. Bear left on path around dog park and sewer pump station building. Turn left on path along other side of Mission Creek.
8. At 4th St. turn right. Continue along UCSF buildings.
9. Continue on 4th St. to 16th St. Turn left and cross 3rd St. to Illinois St.
10. Right on Illinois St. to Mariposa.
11. Left on Mariposa to Terry Francois Blvd. and turn left.
12. Continue on Terry Francois Blvd. past Pier 48.
13. Bear left at China Basin. Continue to 3rd St. at the bridge.
14. Right onto 3rd St.
15. Right onto King Street. If you wish to end your walk here, see bus info above. Otherwise, continue to the Embarcadero and your beginning.

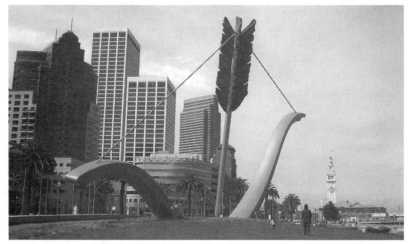

Cupid's Span *Tony Holiday*

workers. As you continue to Townsend and 2nd St. you will see elegant interpretive signposts listing pertinent historic information of San Francisco's early waterfront years. Bloody Thursday occurred in the area from Market to 2nd St. on July 5, 1934, during the International Longshoremen's Workers Union strike, one of the bloodiest union strikes in the country.

> *Walking is the best possible exercise. You should not permit yourself even to think while you walk, but divert yourself by the objects surrounding you.*
> —Thomas Jefferson, in a letter to a friend, 1790

⊿ At South Beach Park, Mark di Suvero's sculpture *Sea Change* stands taller than anything else around. The 700-berth marina has been in operation under Redevelopment Agency management since 1986, and is fully occupied.

⊿ We continue around the marina, past the South Beach Yacht Club, to the AT&T Ball Park that opened in April 2000. It has undergone several name changes. There are sidewalk insets of Giants events in the walkway, but mostly they feature Barry Bonds. The standing room area where people can view the game through the spaces in the fence is democratically run. One is allowed to watch three innings, and then must give his space to another fan.

◢ Continue to 3rd St. to Lefty O'Doul Bridge and cross at the cross-walk. Now we are in the China Basin area named for the China Clippers of the Pacific Mail Steamship Line that docked here at Steamboat Point after the mid-1860s. Walk on the promenade along Mission Creek in front of the dominating China Basin Building. At 4th St. cross at the crosswalk.

◢ But cities move. San Francisco is stretching out toward the south-east, building up parkways and a clean Mission Creek. Along the main streets of King and Townsend and 4th streets, large grocery stores are appearing, bakeries, a special coffeehouse that prepares individual servings of fresh coffee and other sidewalk-front stores. New housing has developed, from condos and low-cost to middle-class rentals. The Mission Bay Branch Library occupies the first floor of the 400-unit senior living center at the corner of King and 4th St.

◢ As you continue, the Mission Creek Marina comes into view. The floating homes are painted in various colors that give a feeling of neighborliness. They are a community of activists, they love living near the water, and they keep it clean; the grounds around their houses have plantings, and many of them also work their garden plots in the community garden.

Embarcadero interpretive panel *Tony Holiday*

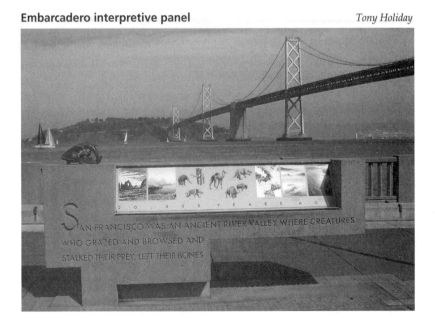

- At the kayak storage building, continue around the sports fields by the volleyball court. Walk left on the path around the dog park and sewer pump station building. At the end of the path, turn left to walk back along the other side of Mission Creek.

- A community garden is on the right. Walk along Channel St. toward the Mission Creek Greenway. This area is slated to be parkland, additional condos, and apartment buildings. Continue through the park to 4th St.

- At 4th St. turn right and continue along an area that was once land occupied by warehouses and a railroad yard and is now the University of California, San Francisco Mission Bay Campus. UCSF began opening laboratories and classrooms on this location in 2003. Several other facilities have opened since that time. The children's and women's specialties and cancer hospital is scheduled to be completed in 2014.

- Continue to 16th St., turn left and cross 3rd St. Walk to Illinois St. and turn right continuing to Mariposa. At Mariposa turn left and continue to Terry Francois Blvd. After turning left on Terry Francois Blvd., continue past The Ramp Restaurant, a very happy place. Everyone enjoys lunching along the water. Then we pass Agua Vista Park, Pier 52 with the historic railroad ferry ramp, the Bayview Boat Club, the new public boat launch ramp the Mariposa/Hunters Point Yacht Club, Pier 50, and Pier 48.

- At the end, to the right is a children's ballpark and Willie McCovey sculpture. Continue left at China Basin Cove, walking along the baseball sculptures, to 3rd St. and right onto King St. to the front entrance of the AT&T Park. The Willie Mayes sculpture is on the right.

- If you wish to end your walk here, check the end of the route for bus service. If not, continue on King St. to the Embarcadero and turn left to your beginning.

- P.S. Yes, level walking is different from stairway walking.

The Blue Greenway

VARIATION 1A

Variation 1A evolved from a walk with a group of Mission Creek residents on the annual bird count around the Mission Creek area. I experienced another aspect of the area—a rich wildlife, camouflaged among the trees and flowers.

1. Begin at the Mission Bay Library at No. 960 4th St. Cross the 4th St. bridge to the south side of Mission Creek. Turn right to walk along the Mission Creek Greenway footpath. The water was clear and we were delighted to see water birds—gulls, coots, western grebes, and mallards. In the trees we were able to see wrentits, white crown sparrows, robins, and chickadees. Overhead we could see double-breasted cormorants.

2. Continue on the footpath along the greenway. The front of the house-boats come into view.

3. Continue past the community garden and turn right. Depending on the season you walk, you will find a huge acacia tree full of yellow allergen blossoms.

4. Walk past the dog park. Bear right and continue past the volleyball court and the kayak storage building.

5. We are walking on the north esplanade in front of the well-designed apartments that consist of low-cost and moderate priced housing and market price condos. Kayakers floated by. We saw bushtits in their nest in one of the bushes along the water. From the back of the floating homes you can see a swan-shaped boat sitting between two of the houses.

6. Continue to 4th St. and turn left to your beginning.

VARIATION 1B

Variation 1B evolved from an amble with an out-of-town guest.

1. Begin on 4th St. across the street from the Mission Bay Library. Walk past Berry St. toward the bridge.

2. Turn left at the esplanade along Mission Creek and the China Basin building.

3. Continue to 3rd St. and the Lefty O'Doul Bridge.

4. Cross 3rd St. at the crosswalk and walk along the back of AT&T Park.

5. Bear left and walk on the Embarcadero.

6. If you feel like continuing to the Ferry Building, it is a treat for all the senses. The interior is an engrossing food encyclopedia. Many of the vendors have samples for you to taste. I bought the candy cap mushroom ice cream. It is extraordinarily delicious.

7. You can end your walk at any point. If you want to continue downtown or to other neighborhoods of the City, there is available transportation.

An Informal Bibliography

Among favorite books that I keep on shelves at eye-level for easy access, I have Doris Muscatine's *Old San Francisco: The Biography of a City from Early Days to the Earthquake* (New York City: G.P. Putnam's Sons, 1975). I enjoy her writing as well as her scholarship. I recommend it without reservation.

Also on my shelves is David Myrick's now out-of-print *San Francisco's Telegraph Hill* (Berkeley: Howell-North Books, 1972). It's a priceless history with archival photographs.

Trustworthy reference books to have on hand are: Gladys Hansen's *San Francisco Almanac* (San Francisco: Chronicle Books, 1995); Judith Lynch Waldhorn and Sally Woodbridge's Victoria's *Legacy: Tours of San Francisco Bay Area Architecture* (San Francisco: 101 Productions, 1978); and William Kostura's *Russian Hill: The Summit, 1853–1906* (San Francisco: Aerie Publications, 1997); Amy Meyer's *New Guardians for the Golden Gate* (Berkeley: UC Press, 2006), a beautifully told story of the 30-year effort of dedicated citizens to save the land for the Golden Gate National Recreation Area; and Doris Sloan's *Geology of the San Francisco Bay Region* (Berkeley: UC Press, 2006).

When writing the St. Francis Wood walk, I found both the following sources invaluable: Mark A. Wilson's "Mason-McDuffie and the Creation of St. Francis Wood," published in *The Argonaut: Journal of the San Francisco Historical Society* (Fall 1997) and Jake Sigg's "New Zealand Christmas Tree," a pamphlet published by Friends of the Urban Forest in August–September 2006.

Randolph Delehanty's *Walks and Tours in the Golden Gate City* (San Francisco: The Dial Press, 1980) is an enlightening, opinionated commentary on the architecture throughout the City.

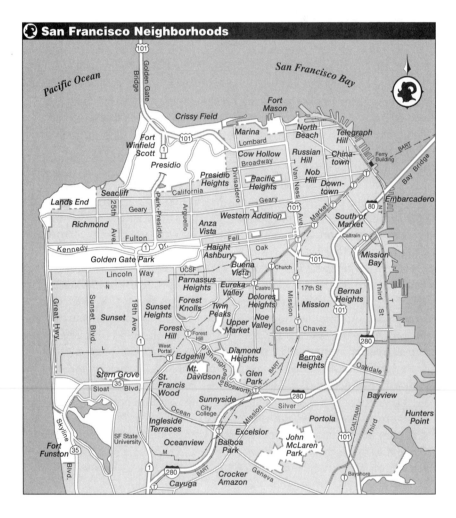

San Francisco Neighborhoods

List of Stairways

There is no such thing as a *complete* anything, but with 670 stairways, this list is rather comprehensive. We have listed all the public stairways *except* stairways that go up to a school, stairways that access private property, and stairways so decrepit they are a danger to traverse. We have marked with an asterisk (*) stairways in problematic neighborhoods. Long stairways that are disconnected by streets are counted as one stairway. Multiple stairways in parks have been listed as one.

No single factor can sum up the character of a stairway. It may be 100 steps but easy (Diamond and 22nd St.), or 30 steps and difficult (Collingwood St.). We have charming stairways (Pemberton) and we have utilitarian stairways (Stonestown). We have elegant concrete stairways (Alta Plaza Park) and we have wood and concrete stairways (Joy). We have stairways bordered by trees, shrubs, flowers, stones, broken glass, railings, Victorian houses, and lean-tos.

Stairways are difficult to push into categories—it seems easier to classify neighborhoods than stairways. Forest Hill and Forest Knolls are unusual in settings and stairways. Golden Gate Heights and Noe Valley have well-designed networks of stairways and retaining walls. Diamond Heights has a series of very long stairways. Telegraph Hill and Russian Hill have alleys and stairways and many houses without street access. Living along the Filbert and Greenwich stairways in the Telegraph Hill area is an incentive to purchase lightweight furniture, like futons. East Bernal Heights has become a forest of stairways, and several intersect community gardens.

Above all, this is a participatory book. The fun is in the walking, in discovering your own variations, and in conversations with neighborhood residents. The exhilarating views are just another bonus of this extraordinary City.

Ratings

My stairway ratings are based on what struck me most during a walk: steepness, length, location, elevation, or beauty—and any combination of these attributes. The slash (/) stands for the word "between."

5   The Scheherazade category. These stairways surprise the walker. Elegant or rustic, short or long, they exhibit variety, stir the imagination, and delight the senses.

4   Impressive qualities with minor shortcomings; one outstanding aspect or extremely attractive section.

3   Little known but deserving of wider recognition because of the environs, human-made or natural. Neighborhood is generally very attractive.

2   Intrinsic to neighborhood history and ambiance. Well-trodden. Functional. In most cases, the architectural context rates considerably higher than the stairway itself, or the view may be worth the visit.

1   It may be so boring that you'll fall asleep on the first landing.

*   An asterisk means that a stairway might be well worth visiting if it were located in a safe neighborhood. This stairway is only for the knowledgeable resident, the wary aficionado.

ANZA VISTA

A neighborhood surrounding the University of San Francisco complex. Small well-kept homes from the 1950s and the Victorian era are part of this area.

RATING

2   **Arbol Lane/Anza Vista & Turk.** Good everyday route.

2   **Arguella/Anza & Edward, into Rossi Recreation Center.** Large granite planter bowls at entrance of two granite stairways.

3   **Blake/Geary & Euclid, into Laurel Hill Playground.** In Laurel Heights.

2   **Cook/Geary & Euclid.** In Laurel Heights. View of Lone Mtn.

2   **Dicha Alley/Lupine & Wood.** Useful and used.

2   **Ewing at Nos. 196–200 to Anza, near Collins.** Ewing Court was a baseball field at one time. Clever.

4   **Lone Mtn., from No. 401 Parker to Beaumont to Stanyan to Rossi.** Long twitton trees, church spires, views of Angel Island and west; nice series of Victorians on McAllister off Parker.

2   **O'Farrell & Lyon.** Rounding a corner.

1   **Sonora Lane/Terra Vista & O'Farrell at No. 90 Terra Vista.**

BALBOA PARK

American Indian street names abound in this neighborhood. Also, it has underground waterways, a creek, and the old Cayuga Lake.

RATING

2   **Alemany, near Rousseau to Mission.**

2   **Balboa Park. San Jose, near Ocean, into park.**

2   **Geneva, near Ocean.** Skyway to City College; stairways midspan to MUNI Metro.

1   **Mission at Trumbull to Alemany.**

2   **Naglee/Alemany & Cayuga.** Across from the most visually stunning Department of Recreation & Park sculpture garden, park, and playground in the City. At head of Cayuga Creek.

2   **Oneida/Alemany & Cayuga.** Practical.

1   **Restani/Restani Way & No. 718 Geneva.** Practical. Only residents know it.

BART AND MUNI METRO STATIONS
RATING

2   **Balboa Park BART-Muni Metro Station at Geneva & San Jose, down into station.**

2   **Civic Center BART Station at 8th & Market, down into station.**

1   **Embarcadero BART-Muni Metro Station at Embarcadero/Market, down into station.** Built in 1973. Concrete stairway and wall, brushed aluminum railings. Interesting edifices of Financial District.

2   **Forest Hill MUNI Metro Station at Laguna Honda, near Dewey, inside station.**

3   **Glen Park BART Station at Diamond/Bosworth & Monterey, down into station.** View. Variety of textures in walks and stairs.

2   **Glen Park BART Station at Monterey at Diamond.** Overcrossing and two stairways down to MUNI Metro stop.

2   **Market. Castro MUNI Metro Station at Castro & Market, down into station.**

3   **Market. Church at Market, down into MUNI Metro Station.** Terrazzo stairway, ceramic tile walls.

3   **Mission. 16th St. BART Station at Mission, down into station.**

3   **Mission. 24th St. BART Station at Mission, down into station.**

3   **Montgomery BART-Muni Metro Station at Montgomery & Market, down into station.** In the Financial District among historic and non-historic highrises. Bubbled tile wall.

4   **Powell BART-Muni Metro Station at Powell & Market, down into station.** Wide esplanade into Hallidie Plaza, near visitors information center. Unimaginative.

2   **Van Ness MUNI Metro Station at Van Ness & Market, down into station.**

2   **West Portal MUNI Metro Station at West Portal & Santa Clara, down into station.**

BAYVIEW

This neighborhood has some historic buildings.

RATING

*   **Bayview Park.** All concrete. Two sets of old stone stairs near summit. Hidden.
*   **Gilroy & Jamestown.**
*   **Hawes & Innes.**
*   **Hilltop Park. Lillian at Beatrice, up to park.**
*   **Hilltop Park. LaSalle at Osceola, up to park.** Largest sundial in state.
*   **Key/3rd St. & Bayview Park entrance.** Six small stairways from street to sidewalk.
*   **Key at Jennings.** Sidewalk stairs.
*   **Lane to No. 1501 Lower LaSalle.**
*   **LaSalle to Health Center/Osceola & Garlington Court.** Wood stairway.
*   **LaSalle & Osceola to Health Center.**
*   **LaSalle-Upper LaSalle to Lindsay Circle.**
*   **Mini-Park at Lillian & Rosie Lee Lane.**
*   **Quesada/Newhall & 3rd Street.**
*   **Quesada-Upper Quesada to Lower Quesada, near Newhall.**
*   **Revere/Newhall & 3rd St. Sidewalk stairway.**
*   **Thornton/3rd St. & Latona.** Sidewalk stairway on both sides.

BERNAL HEIGHTS

A neighborhood mix of professionals, blue-collar workers, and artists. Most stairways have adjoining gardens.

RATING

4   **Andover/Powhattan & Bernal Heights Park.** Defies description. Homespun array and diversity. View.

1   **Appleton/San Jose & Mission.** Utilitarian.

2   **Aztec/Aztec & Shotwell.**

3   **Banks/Chapman & Powhattan.** Concrete and new wood stairway.

2   **Bernal Heights Park. Coso, near Bonview, into park.** Trail and wood stairway.

2   **Bernal Heights Park. End of Esmeralda Stwy. up to trail, into park.**

3   **Bernal Heights Park. Across street from 39 Ellsworth into park.** Nine cobblestone steps connect to trail. View.

3   **Bessie/Bessie & Mirabel at Shotwell.** Narrow, unexpected. Half-sized lots on Bessie.

4   **Brewster/Brewster at Costa & Upper Brewster & Rutledge.** Concrete up to Dogpatch Community Garden. Wood stairway up through poplars. Two community gardens accessed from this stairway.

2   **Bronte, uphill from Cortland, south.**

1   **Bronte/Tompkins & Jarboe.** Practical, railroad ties.

3   **Chapman to Powhattan at Nevada.** New wood stairway. Walking up and down slope through driveways difficult.

2   **Coso/Prospect & Winfield.** View. Cars from private driveways have to cross the stairs.

2   **Cuvier/San Jose & Bosworth.**

5   **Esmeralda/Coleridge & Bernal Heights Park.** Three separate stairways, along right of way, crossing Lundys Lane, Prospect, Winfield, and Elsie. Three blocks of gardens.

3   **Esmeralda/Brewster & Franconia.** Elevated above landscaped hillside. Timber and concrete; benches and lighting. Views.

1   **Esmeralda-Upper Esmeralda to Lower Esmeralda at Peralta.** Wood stairway.

4   **Eugenia/Prospect & Winfield.** Among trees.

1   **Eve Stwy./Upper & Lower Holladay at Wright & Peralta.** A wraith of itself.

3   **Fair Stwy./Coleridge & Prospect.** Grove of trees at top. Views.

3   **Faith/Brewster & Holladay.**

4   **Franconia/Franconia & Brewster Stwy.** Enter on Franconia at sign. Nice neighborhood community garden, 1991. Railroad-tie stairway, through Dogpatch Community Garden. View toward Bay & Hunters Point.

3   **Franconia/Mullen & Montcalm.** Wood, short. Shrubbery and trees alongside. View.

3   **Franconia/Mullen & Peralta.** Concrete, wood, landscaped.

3   **Franconia/Montcalm & Rutledge.** New stairway. Neighborhood project.

4 **Gates/Bernal Heights Blvd. & Powhattan.** Pressure-treated wood timbers; native plants on slope; planter boxes at base. Easy walking on stairs.

3 **Harrison/Ripley & Norwich.** Wood and concrete stairway, benches, lighting. Great view of downtown. Egger Open Space garden. Builder/subdivider put in stairway.

1 **Highland to San Jose.** Hefty.

4 **Holladay/Peralta & Bayshore.** View the link between an isolated, urban neighborhood and the main traffic arteries north and south.

2 **Holly Park. Boscana at Holly Park Circle, into park.**

2 **Holly Park. Highland at Holly Park Circle, into park.**

2 **Holly Park. Murray at Holly Park Circle, into park.**

2 **Holly Park. Across from Junipero Serra School at Holly Park Circle.**

2 **Holly Park. East side up from Highland, in park.**

5 **Joy/Holladay & Brewster.** Rural. New wood stairway and benches. Existing gardens to be preserved.

3 **Kingston/Coleridge & Prospect.** Semblance of floating stairs. Railing. Long footpath and rock formation alongside.

2 **Manchester at end of street below Bernal Heights Park.**

3 **Mayflower/Holladay & Franconia.** Wood stairway, trees—maytens, oak, and purple leaf plum.

3 **Mayflower/Bradford & Carver.** Short wood stairways lead to wood chip path. Garden flagstone marker.

5 **Mirabel at No. 11 to Percita.** Hidden. Extremely narrow.

2 **Montcalm/Wright & Peralta.** Rustic; through garden.

3 **Montezuma at Coso to Mirabel.** Cuts a corner.

3 **Moultrie/Bernal Heights Blvd. & Powhattan.** Concrete plus footpath. Truly hidden and rural. Plantings alongside. First decisive victory of the American Revolution was at Fort Moultrie, S.C., in 1776.

2 **Mullen Stwy., next to No. 146, near Franconia.** Concrete. Goes up to Peralta Point Open Space. Extraordinary views.

4 **Ogden/Nevada & Prentiss.** Through community gardens.

2 **Peralta Point Open Space/Montcalm & Mullen.** Wood stairway.

2 **Peralta/Rutledge & Montcalm.**

4 **Peralta/Samoset & Rutledge.** Magnificent gardens, extraordinary views.

2 **Powhattan/Gates & Ellsworth.** Short wood stairway leads to a path.

4 **Prentiss/Bernal Heights Blvd. & Powhattan.** Prentiss to Chapman, wood timber; native plants on slope; two short angled concrete stairways at Powhattan. Easy walking.

2   **Prospect/Cortland & Santa Maria.**

1   **Richland to San Jose.** Hefty.

3   **Rosenkrantz/Bernal Heights Blvd. & Bernal Heights Blvd. at Powhattan.** Wood stairway to auto/foot path. Left to wood and concrete stairways.

4   **Rutledge/Holladay, Mullen, Brewster, & Wolf Patch Community Garden.** Pedestrian path. Wide neighborhood use.

3   **Tompkins/Putnam & Nevada.** View of industrial side of the City.

3   **Virginia/Eugenia & Winfield.** Part of a series of three separate stairways from retaining wall to lower level. Some stairways dead end.

BUENA VISTA (CORONA HEIGHTS)

An old neighborhood with large mansions and converted flats.

RATING

3   **Alpine/Waller & Duboce.** Sidewalk stairway.

4   **Buena Vista East. Baker & Haight, into Buena Vista Park.**

2   **Buena Vista East. At Buena Vista Blvd. Nos. 75–101, 95, 135, 351, 437, into Buena Vista Park.** Short wood stairways.

5   **Buena Vista East. Buena Vista Blvd. at Nos. 355–399, into Buena Vista Park.** Terraced stairways.

5   **Buena Vista East. Buena Vista Terrace & Duboce, into Buena Vista Park.** Ornament above entrance wall gives unusual effect. Curving steps. View.

3   **Buena Vista East. Park Hill, into Buena Vista Park.** Concrete, wide stairway.

4   **Buena Vista East. Waller/Broderick & Buena Vista at No. 101.** Sidewalk stairway, easy risers. View of Mt. Diablo.

5   **Buena Vista East. Waller/Broderick, into Buena Vista Park.** Garrett Eckbo was the architect of Buena Vista Park erosion-control measures, which include stairways. Work in progress. Hidden. View.

5   **Buena Vista East & Buena Vista West at Upper Terrace.** Boardwalk accommodates strollers and handicap to the summit.

2   **Buena Vista West. Central, into Buena Vista Park.** Stone stairway.

3   **Buena Vista West. Frederick, into Buena Vista Park.** Concrete, wide. Should be extended.

4   **Buena Vista West. Haight/Central & Lyon, into Buena Vista Park. Lovely.** One of the early, beautiful San Francisco neighborhoods.

4   **Buena Vista West. Java, into Buena Vista Park.** Wood stairway.

3   **Buena Vista West. Lyon & Haight, into Buena Vista Park.**

4   **Buena Vista West. Welland Lathrop Memorial Walk, into Buena Vista Park, across from No. 547 Buena Vista West.** Pine trees, view. Lathrop was one of the early modern dance teachers in San Francisco.

2   **Buena Vista West. Buena Vista Blvd. Nos. 555 & 737, into Buena Vista Park.** Wood stairways.

3   **Buena Vista Park.** Stone stairway on summit. Part of 400-mile Bay Area Ridge Trail. Wood stairways within park lead to paved paths, boardwalk, and summit.

4   **Corona Heights Park.** New series of wood stairways, new plantings by Native Plant Society. Surrounds Randall Museum.

3   **DeForest/Beaver & Flint.** A stairway street, 3 feet wide and 125 feet long, built around 1913. At the top is Corona Heights Park.

3   **Duboce/Castro & Divisadero.** South side. Special. Very steep.

3   **Duboce/Divisadero & Alpine.** North side. Shallow steps. 25% grade.

4   **Henry Stwy./No. 473 Roosevelt & Castro.** Hidden cul-de-sac. A definite charmer.

CHINATOWN

A special combination of sounds, smells, and colors.

RATING

5   **California/opposite No. 660, into St. Mary's Square.** A relatively low-rated stairway in a fascinating locale.

2   **Grant & Bush Stwy. & Chinatown Gate.** Entrance to Chinatown. Just enough of a lift into another world.

5   **Portsmouth Square. Clay/Kearny & Walter Lum Pl.**

5   **Portsmouth Square. Interior of square toward Kearny.**

5   **Portsmouth Square. Kearny & Clay.**

5   **Portsmouth Square. Kearny & Washington.**

5   **Portsmouth Square. Walter Lum Pl./Clay & Washington.**

5   **Portsmouth Square. Washington & Walter Lum Pl.**

DIAMOND HEIGHTS

A neighborhood of views, hills, and canyons.

RATING

4   **Coralino/No. 289 Amber to No. 92 Cameo.** Woodsy. White-crowned sparrows love it.

2   **Diamond Heights Blvd. & No. 5411, into Walter Haas Park.**

5 **Glen Canyon Park to George Christopher Park, Crags Court, Berkeley Way.** Log and plank, and rock stairways on several trails. Paths with rock formation and flowers.

4 **Gold Mine & No. 98 to Douglass & No. 681 28th St.** Concrete path, with stairway to start.

5 **Gold Mine at No. 160/Ora & Jade (Opalo).** Stairway access to Christopher Park. Christopher Park is next to the Diamond Heights shopping center.

5 **Onique/No. 101 Berkeley & No. 289 Berkeley & No. 400 Gold Mine & No. 243 Topaz.** Three separate stairways. Forty-five-degree view of San Francisco. Surroundings of eucalyptus, pine, canyons, and hummingbirds. A four-tiered Chinese hopscotch walk.

2 **Safira Lane/27th St. at No. 881 & Diamond Heights Blvd. at Nos. 5173 & 5147, adjoining Douglass Playground.** Part of a long stairway outlined by trees. Nice access.

3 **Turquoise/No. 48 & No. 52.** Goes to Amber & down to Glen Canyon Park. Gardens.

DOLORES HEIGHTS

A lovely, hilly neighborhood in the Mission District.

RATING

2 **Cumberland/Church & Dolores Park.**

5 **Cumberland/Noe No. 670 & Sanchez.** Very impressive.

4 **Cumberland/Sanchez & Church.** View. Hidden. Additional curving ramp and wall. Dense vegetation.

3 **Dolores Park.** On walkway across park connecting to 19th St.

3 **Dolores Park. 19th St./Church & Dolores Park, over MUNI Metro tracks.** Three separate stairways into park.

2 **Hancock/Church & Dolores Park.**

5 **Liberty/Noe & Rayburn.** Beautifully designed foliage plantings. Art Moderne houses alongside. View to east and west.

4 **Liberty/Sanchez & Church.** Inviting area with lots of foliage. Two stairways connecting Upper and Lower Liberty.

2 **Sanchez/Cumberland & Sanchez Stwy.** Sidewalk stairways on both sides.

4 **Sanchez/19th St. & Cumberland.** City-designed entrance stairway, plus sidewalk stairs. At top, four large 60-year-old cypresses alongside. View.

5 **Sanchez/Liberty & 21st St.** Network of stairs, one of the most beautiful series in the City. View.

5 **20th St. & Noe.** Impressive. Backdrop of high curving wall.

5 **20th St. & Sanchez.** Two stairways at top connecting to one stairway. Views. Enter a street that connects with Noe stairway and ramp.

3 **21st St./Castro & Collingwood.**

3 **22nd St./Castro & Collingwood.** Profuse plantings.

4 **22nd St./Diamond & Collingwood.** Greenery all around.

4 **22nd St./Church & Vicksburg.** Sidewalk stairways on both sides of street. If you feel you're sliding backward, it's because the steps slope backward. One of the steepest climbs in the city.

DOWNTOWN

A neighborhood subject to significant changes.

RATING

2 **Stockton Tunnel/Sutter & Bush and Sacramento & California.** Stairways utilitarian and unimaginative.

4 **Union Square. Powell & Geary, into square.** Wide corner stairway. Magicians, music, skits, and street artists—lots of local color. Popular with San Franciscans.

3 **Union Square. Powell & Post, into square.** Walkway and short corner stairway.

4 **Union Square. Stockton & Geary, into square.** Wide corner stairway with staggered steps.

3 **Union Square. Stockton & Post, into square.** Short stairways at corner.

3 **Union Square. Multiple stairways on Post, Stockton, & Geary/Stockton & Powell and Geary & Post.**

EDGEHILL

The steepness of the hill limits the number of homes on this street, which winds up to the summit.

RATING

3 **Dorchester to Kensington. Crosses Allston & Granville.** Concrete path leading to stairways at Granville.

3 **Edgehill Open Space.** Wood stairway leads to No. 60 Shangri La Way.

2 **Garcia/Edgehill Way & Idora, connecting Upper and Lower Garcia.** Two stairways.

2 **Garcia/Vasquez & Edgehill Way, connecting Upper and Lower Garcia.** Brick. Quaint.

2	**Idora/Garcia & Laguna Honda, connecting Upper and Lower Idora.**
1	**Lennox, opposite No. 146.** Street up to tennis courts.
5	**Pacheco/Merced & Vasquez.** Echoes the Grand Stairway to the north.
2	**Ulloa at Waithman.** Sidewalk steps to street.
3	**Ulloa/Kensington & Waithman.** Twenty-five small stairways between street and sidewalk.
2	**West Portal Drive & No. 21.** Alley and stairs in rear.

EMBARCADERO

Area has been revitalized. The Farmers' Market at the Ferry Building is one of the most popular attractions in the City.

5	**Commercial/Sansome & No. 1 Embarcadero Center.** Sculpture at entrance; concentric circle of tiles in pavement carry forward the visual pattern throughout the Embarcadero Center and Hyatt Regency Hotel. See sculpture and gardens throughout center.
2	**Embarcadero Center.** Multiple levels with stairways into and within center.
2	**Ferry Building at North End Plaza.** Wide stairway.
3	**Justin Herman Plaza at end of Market & Embarcadero.** Plaza-scale steps for walking or watching. Action and palm trees. Two narrow stairs to lookouts in midst of Vaillancourt Fountain.
4	**Maritime Plaza/Washington/Clay/Battery/Front & Davis.** Six sets of stairways. Open space.
2	**Pacific/Battery & Sansome, into Masto Plaza.**

EUREKA VALLEY

This neighborhood has a community organization active since 1881, a large gay population, fine Victorians, beautiful gardens, and the Castro—a movie palace built in 1922.

1	**Acme Alley/Corwin No. 95 & Grand View.** Wood and red brick stairway at Grand View with steep path to Corwin. Stone path from Corwin to Seward.
3	**Caselli/Clayton & Market.**
3	**Clover Lane/No. 101 Caselli & No. 4612 19th St. Cross alley and continue up.** Variety of stairs—plaster, concrete, railroad-tie and concrete,

with partially covered bowl-shaped steps. Top of stairway between Nos. 4612 & 4608 19th St.

2   **Dixie/No. 3801 Market & No. 285 Grand View near Alvarado.**

4   **Douglass at Corwin.** Street to upper level. One of our favorite corners of the City.

3   **Douglass at No. 414/Corwin & Romain.** Street to upper level. Profuse plantings.

3   **Douglass at Romain.** Street to upper level. Profuse plantings.

1   **Douglass at 19th St.**

4   **Douglass/20th St. & Corwin.** Delightful discovery. Trees alongside. Exceptional.

1   **Douglass at 24th St., into Noe Valley Park.**

2   **Grand View to Market, near Grand View Terrace.**

3   **Grand View to Stanton at Market.** Hidden. An archaeological find.

3   **Mono/Market & Eagle, with a ramp to Caselli.** A long twitton.

3   **19th St. at No. 4612 to Kite Hill.** Rustic stairs and path along Upper Clover Lane.

2   **Prosper/16th St. & Pond.** Behind Eureka branch library—an inviting place, a fine book collection.

3   **Seward at Douglass & No. 31 Seward.** Stairways connecting to raised sidewalk. Enriches street by adding another level of viewing. Also very useful. Imaginative choice of plants. Beautiful corner of the City.

2   **Seward at No. 30.** One stairway into Seward Playground, two within it.

4   **Short/Market & Yukon.**

1   **Upper Market Walkway/Glendale & Romain.** Short stairway.

3   **Yukon/Eagle & Short.** Railroad-tie stairway into Kite Hill Park.

EXCELSIOR (McLAREN PARK)

A stable neighborhood of diverse ethnic groups. Stairways reminiscent of the everyday kind of European towns.

RATING

2   **Athens/Avalon & Peru.**

2   **Crocker-Amazon Park. Geneva, opposite No. 1572, into park.**

3   **Crocker-Amazon Park. Prague, near Russia, into park.** Wood and concrete.

2   **Crocker-Amazon Playground Skate Park to McLaren Park.** Hidden in northeast corner of playground.

2 **Kenney Alley at No. 646 London to Mission.** Difficult to find.

1 **Lisbon/Russia & France.** Seventeen stairways between sidewalk and street levels.

3 **McLaren Park. Ervine at Wilde.** Asphalt path to stairway. View at top.

2 **McLaren Park. Excelsior at No. 1021, near Munich, into park.**

2 **McLaren Park. LaGrande & Brazil, into park.**

2 **McLaren Park. On the path/Lake McNab & Shelley Dr.** Railroad-tie stairway.

2 **McLaren Park. On the path/Shelley Lake & Shelley Dr.** Railroad-tie stairway.

3 **McLaren Park. Prague at Brazil, into park.**

2 **McLaren Park. Prague at Excelsior, into park.**

2 **McLaren Park. University at Woolsey, into park.** Wood stairway.

2 **McLaren Park. Yale, into park.**

4 **Munich/Ina & Excelsior.** Hidden. View. Built in 1977.

4 **Peru/Athens & Valmar.** Aggregate and railroad ties, designed by R. Schadt. Great views.

2 **Sunglow Lane/Gladstone & Silver at Oxford.**

FOREST HILL

The City accepted responsibility for maintaining the non-regulation streets of this neighborhood.

RATING

4 **Alton/No. 60 Ventura to No. 70 Alton & No. 400 Lower Pacheco.**

4 **Alton/Lower Pacheco to No. 399 Upper Pacheco, continuing to No. 60 Sotelo.**

4 **Castenada at No. 140 to Pacheco at No. 334.** Adjacent is a Maybeck house with delightful details, like the carved grapevines along the eaves.

2 **Castenada, opposite No. 249.** Stairs to nowhere.

2 **Dorantes & San Marcos.** Rounding a corner. Street to sidewalk.

2 **Dorantes & Magellan.** Two corner stairways and one at No. 320 Magellan.

5 **8th Ave. at No. 1998 to No. 20 Ventura.**

2 **Forest Hill MUNI Metro Station, to Magellan.**

5 **Montalvo/Castenada at No. 376 to San Marcos to 9th Ave. to Mendosa.** Variety in terrain and architecture. Four separate "custom-made" stairways.

| 2 | **Murphy Playground/9th Ave. & 8th Ave., near Pacheco.** Seven separate stairways. |

| 5 | **Pacheco/Magellan & No. 249 Castenada.** Grandest and most elegant of all San Francisco stairways. |

| 2 | **Pacheco-Upper Pacheco at No. 364 to Lower Pacheco.** |

| 5 | **Santa Rita at No. 60 to Upper and Lower San Marcos.** A unique three-way stairway. |

| 2 | **12th Ave. (at end) to Dorantes.** Stairway and a long path. |

FOREST KNOLLS

A neighborhood heavily forested with eucalyptus.

| 4 | **Ashwood Lane/Clarendon & Warren at No. 101.** Among the trees. View across to Mt. Davidson. |

| 4 | **Blairwood Lane/No. 113 Warren & No. 95 & No. 101 Crestmont.** Three separate stairways. View. With green railings, it's almost camouflaged among pine and acacia. Floating stairs. Surreal view of TV tower. |

| 2 | **Forest Knolls Stwy. at No. 191 Forest Knolls Drive, in cul-de-sac, down to school playground.** |

| 3 | **Glenhaven Lane/Oak Park & No. 191 Christopher.** |

| 5 | **Oakhurst Lane/Warren & Crestmont.** View of ocean. Difficult. Longest continuous stairway to highest elevation in San Francisco. Eucalyptus forest. |

FORT FUNSTON

Part of Golden Gate National Recreation Area. Off Hwy. 35, south of zoo.

| 4 | **"Horsetail" Stwy., left of parking lot.** Down along Pliocene-age cliffs, to ocean shore. Plan trip for low tide. Great view of hang-gliding activity. |

| 2 | **John Muir Drive at Skyline, on path to Fort Funston.** |

| 1 | **Multiple stairways at gunnery and battery sites in Fort Funston.** |

FORT MASON

Magnificent example of conversion from military fort to part of the Golden Gate National Recreation Area.

RATING

2   **Alcatraz Island.** Some stairways public, most private.

2   **Aquatic Park Promenade & Upper Railroad-Tie Walkway/Polk & Van Ness.**

4   **Fort Mason. Black Point Battery to Aquatic Park.** View.

2   **Fort Mason. Black Point Battery to top of wall.** Wood stairway.

3   **Fort Mason. Black Point Gunnery behind San Francisco International Youth Hostel.** Four stairways around gunnery and one on side of entrance below.

2   **Fort Mason. Community Garden.** Three stone and wood stairways within garden.

3   **Fort Mason. End of Franklin to Black Point Battery & picnic area.**

3   **Fort Mason. Great Meadow & Bldg. E at Pier 3.**

3   **Fort Mason. Great Meadow & San Francisco International Youth Center near Bufano *Peace* sculpture.**

4   **Jefferson/Beach, Hyde & Larkin. Amphitheater in Victoria Park.**

FORT WINFIELD SCOTT

A fort within the Presidio. Beautiful rock walls, stairs, and vegetation.

RATING

5   **Batteries to Bluffs/Langdon & Marshall Beach & Baker Beach.** Multiple wood stairways along the ocean.

4   **Kobbe, opposite No. 1324 to tennis practice area.**

4   **Kobbe, opposite No. 1328 to tennis courts.**

4   **Kobbe, opposite No. 1330, at parking area to recreation hall.** Rock walls along stairways.

1   **Multiple stairways at gunnery and battery sites in Fort Scott.**

3   **Native Plant Garden, to upper nursery.**

2   **Ruckman/Appleton & Ralston. Left sidewalk stairway.**

2   **Tennis courts: Multiple stairways into and around.**

4   **Wool Court & Upton, opposite No. 1337 Pope sign to tennis courts parking lot.** Curving with stone work along sides.

5   **Wool Court & Upton intersection.** First-rate stone footbridge and stairways.

GLEN PARK

Cows roamed the meadowland in this neighborhood in the 1880s.

3 **Amatista Lane/Bemis, near Miguel to Everson.** Hardy. Along Fairmount Plaza.

2 **Bemis, Nos. 130 & 134 at Mateo.** Stairs along Bemis up to sidewalk.

3 **Billy Goat Hill.** Three log stairways to top of hill.

2 **Burnside at Bosworth, across from No. 1035 Bosworth.**

2 **Chilton at Bosworth, across from No. 907 Bosworth.** Long ramp with four stairs at bottom.

2 **Diamond & Moffit.**

2 **Glen Canyon Park. Bosworth at No. 1231, into park.**

3 **Glen Canyon Park. Elk at Sussex, into park.** Railroad ties.

3 **Glen Canyon Park to George Christopher Park, Crags Court, Berkeley Way.** Various wood stairways on several trails.

2 **Glen Park Village Garden. Diamond at No. 2783, into garden.**

2 **Hamerton/Bosworth & Mangels.**

5 **Harry Stwy. at No. 190 Beacon to Laidley.** Unusual stairway that connects to Noe Valley, Glen Park, and Diamond Heights, too. Secluded. Built in 1932 by contractor Easton & Smith.

1 **Penny Lane/Diamond at Castro.** Convenient, with few steps.

1 **Roanoke/San Jose & Arlington.** A walker's solution to freeway divisiveness.

2 **St. Mary's/San Jose & Arlington at No. 439.** Hidden.

GOLDEN GATE HEIGHTS

Carl Larsen, from Denmark, deeded this acreage to the City in 1928.

4 **Aerial Way/14th Ave. & Funston.** Very long trek upward.

3 **Aerial Way/No. 475 Ortega & No. 801 Pacheco.** Long. Ice plants stabilize soil. Part of a network of stairways, all rated 4 or 5.

2 **Aloha & Lomita.** Corner connecting stairway.

5 **Cascade Walk/Ortega, Pacheco, & Funston.** Secluded. Special.

2 **8th Ave./Moraga & Lawton.** Twelve small stairways between street and sidewalk.

2 **Fanning & 14th Ave.** Rounding a corner.

2 **Fanning & 15th Ave.**

4   **15th Ave./Kirkham & Lawton.** Pine trees alongside. Walk up slowly.

1   **15th Ave., near Fanning & Quintara.** Street to sidewalk stairway.

2   **15th Ave., near Moraga to Upper 15th.**

2   **Golden Gate Heights Park. Radio & 12th Ave.** Railroad-tie-stairway. Precarious.

5   **Golden Gate Heights Park. 12th Ave. & Cragmont, into park to tennis courts.** Cobblestone stairways.

3   **Golden Gate Heights Park. 12th Ave. at playground, to tennis courts.**

4   **Grand View Park. 14th Ave. to the top of park.** Eucalyptus, wood stairway, and views.

4   **Grand View Park. Upper 15th Ave. to the top of park.** Wood stairway, wood handrails, and concrete piers.

3   **Grand View Park.** Log stairways at top of park and northside.

4   **Mandalay Lane/No. 2001 14th Ave. & 15th Ave. & Pacheco.** Ocean view.

5   **Moraga/15th & 16th Aves.** Ceramic tile stairway. Children call it the "magic stairway."

5   **Moraga/Funston & top of Grand View Park.** Three stairways.

4   **Mount/No. 1795 14th Ave. & No. 1798 15th Ave.**

2   **9th Ave./Lawton & Moraga.** Fourteen small stairways between street and sidewalk.

4   **Noriega to 15th Ave. & Sheldon Terrace.** Huge rock outcropping.

4   **Oriole Way/Pacheco & Cragmont.** Lots of foliage and long landings.

4   **Ortega Way/14th Ave. & No. 1894 15th Ave.** Very long and very practical. Ocean view. Ice plants on sides.

4   **Pacheco & 12th Ave.** Curving a corner. Community garden.

2   **Pacheco & 14th Ave.** Rounding a corner.

4   **Pacheco/14th & 15th Ave.** View.

3   **Pacheco & 16th Ave.** Rounding a corner.

4   **Quintara at No. 500/14th and 15th Aves.** Great sunset viewing area. Double stairway a third of the way. Built in 1928. View.

3   **Quintara & 16th Ave.** Nice curving wide-rounded corner.

5   **Selma Way/No. 477 Noriega & No. 564 Ortega.** View. High, high, high.

3   **16th Ave./Kirkham & Lawton.** Stairway built before the surrounding houses.

3   **16th Ave./Pacheco & Quintara.** Series of small stairways. Graceful.

GOLDEN GATE PARK

Stairs are still being built here.

RATING

5   **AIDS Memorial.** Curved pathways and stairways.

3   **Anglers Lodge, off JFK Drive, opposite buffalo paddock.** Stone stairway.

2   **Big Recreation area. Street to tennis courts.** Wood stairway and a stone stairway.

3   **Botanical Gardens-Arboretum/Martin Luther King Drive & 9th Ave.** Minimum 18 stairways. Variety of materials: log, plank, tree root, wood, stone, concrete, and stone slab. Some stones date back to 1188, and were brought from the Cistercian Monastery in Madrid, Spain, by William Randolph Hearst.

2   **Children's Playground.** Wood stairway down to merry-go-round.

3   **Children's Playground to Kezar Court.** Curved stone stairway.

4   **Conservatory of Flowers. To walkway and front entrance from lawn area.** Wide concrete stairway.

3   **Conservatory of Flowers. Right side, east to Daliha Gardens.** Concrete stairway.

3   **Fulton at Arguello.** Curving railroad-tie stairs and sides. Most of sides covered.

2   **Fulton at 6th Ave.** Railroad-tie stairs.

3   **Fulton at 10th Ave.** Wide railroad-tie and blacktop stairway. Into play and rest area. Designed by Walter Kocian.

3   **Horseshoe Court near Conservatory Drive East & Arguello.** Stone stairway. Built in the 1930s.

2   **Japanese Tea Garden/Back of garden & east side of Stow Lake.** Wide stone stairway leading to walkway.

1   **JFK Drive: Up to restrooms past buffalo paddock.** Street to sidewalk.

3   **JFK Drive: Down to Chain of Lakes, north side.**

3   **JFK Drive: Intersection of Bernice Rogers Way & JFK Drive.** Wood stairway. Leads to footpath.

2   **Lincoln at 7th Ave., into Golden Gate Park.** Log and plank stairway.

2   **Martin Luther King Drive. Murphy Windmill & Great Highway.** Wood stairway. Continues to footpath at upper level.

2   **Martin Luther King Drive. Street to Stow Lake.** Concrete stairway.

2   **Martin Luther King Drive. West at 19th Ave.** Log stairway.

2   **Martin Luther King Drive. Baseball court at 7th Ave.** Concrete stairway.

4   Stanyan/Haight & Waller, into Golden Gate Park. Concrete with multiple landings.

3   Stow Lake. Huntington Falls/Stow Lake Shore and top of Strawberry Hill. Railroad-tie and chicken-wire boxes filled with boulders and stones. A stairway for giants, and a giant waterfall.

5   Stow Lake. Strawberry Hill/Stow Lake Shore and top of hill at bridge. Fine view. Built of railroad ties, will connect with two stairways, one on each side of Huntington Falls.

2   Stow Lake. To Strawberry Hill/Chinese Pavilion & Falls Stairway. Stone stairway.

HAIGHT ASHBURY

Deliberate remains of the 1960s counterculture in Lower Haight. Upper Haight is a stable community of professionals and middle class families. Beautiful Victorians.

2   Clayton/Frederick & Carl. Stairway down into Richard Gamble Memorial Park.

5   Frederick & Carl/Arguello & Willard, opposite Kezar Stadium. Parkview Commons. Five sets of stairways, with various patterns, surrounded by foliage, trees, and bushes.

2   Frederick at Willard. Ceremonial steps down to colonnaded entry to Kezar Stadium.

INGLESIDE TERRACE

Well-planned community, west of Twin Peaks and near San Francisco State University, with curved streets. Developed by Joseph Leonard around 1913. Famous for its large sundial and early racetrack.

2   Alemany & Head St., near Palmetto. Rebuilt in 2005.

2   Alemany, opposite Victoria. Goes down into dog park. New in 2005.

3   San Leandro at No. 344/Moncado & Ocean.

2   Shakespeare/Shakespeare & DeLong.

2   Worcester, near Alemany. Goes down to shopping center.

3   Wyton/19th Ave. & Junipero Serra. Footpath with stairway at each end.

LANDS END

Great area for ocean breezes and beaches.

3 **Coastal Trail to El Camino Del Mar Trail, just below the VA Hospital.**

4 **Coastal Trail.** Short Peeler-core stairway at El Camino Del Mar Trail; one long and four shorter stairways at Painted Rock Cliff and Dead Man's Point.

3 **Multiple Stairways.** Two wood stairways/parking lot and El Camino Del Mar; two stairways/trailhead to Point Lobos Overlook.

2 **Eagle's Point at El Camino Del Mar.** Wood stairway up to viewing platform near road.

3 **El Camino Del Mar Trail/back of Palace of Legion of Honor & USS *San Francisco* Naval Memorial.**

5 **Mile Rock Stwy./Coastal Trail & Mile Rock Beach.** Leads to Lands End and Maze.

5 **Sutro Baths Stwy./Merrie Way parking lot & Sutro Baths.** Railroad-tie stairway.

4 **USS *San Francisco* Naval Memorial Stwy./48th Ave & El Camino Del Mar to the Coastal Trail.**

MARINA

Development of this neighborhood was given impetus from the 1915 International Exposition.

2 **Bay St./Webster & Buchanan, into George Moscone Recreation Center.**

2 **Crissy Field entrance to St. Francis Yacht Club at Lyon, to benches and to water.**

3 **Wave Organ at end of jetty by Golden Gate Yacht Club, around structure and down to water.**

MISSION

One of the largest districts in San Francisco. Divided into more than a dozen sub-neighborhoods.

3 **Franklin Square. Bryant at 16th St., into square.**

3 **Franklin Square. Bryant at 17th St., into square.**

3   **Franklin Square. 17th St./Bryant & Potrero, into square.**

1   **Garfield Square. Harrison at 25th & 26th Sts., into square.**

1   **Garfield Square. Harrison/25th & 26th Sts., into square.**

1   **Garfield Square. Treat at 26th St., into square.**

2   **25th St./Fair Oaks & Dolores.** Sidewalk stairway. Faint concrete treads like railroad ties.

MT. DAVIDSON

A neighborhood circling the highest elevation in San Francisco (938′). The cross and the surrounding plateau are now privately owned. Be cautious. Fog can make the stairways wet.

RATING

2   **Acova Alley/No. 219 Bella Vista Way at 550 Myra, opposite Dorcas Way.** Stairway beside Miraloma School.

3   **Burlwood & Los Palmos.** Rounding a corner.

3   **Casitas at Cresta Vista.** Rounding a corner.

2   **Chaves & Del Sur.** Seven-step corner-cutter.

2   **Globe Alley at No. 96 Cresta Vista to Hazelwood, near Los Palmos.** Combination easement and stairway.

2   **Hazelwood & Los Palmos.** Rounding a corner.

2   **Lulu Alley/Los Palmos & No. 450 to No. 500 Melrose.** Combination easement and stairway.

3   **Malta/Upper Malta No. 11 and Lower Malta No. 50.** Colorful garden.

3   **Mangels/Brentwood & Melrose.** Stairway down from elevated driveway curving corner.

2   **Marietta-Upper Marietta at No. 466 to Lower Marietta.**

2   **Melrose at Mangels & Ridgewood.** Corner cutter.

2   **Miraloma at No. 2 to Portola.**

4   **Mt. Davidson. Juanita Way at No. 275 Juanita, near Marne.** Fog, moss, stone, and fresh air. Red rocks and cobblestone treads lead up onto Mt. Davidson. Nature trail. Pine and eucalyptus.

3   **Mt. Davidson. Rockdale Drive, next to Nos. 919 and 925.** Cobblestone stairs into forest trails on Mt. Davidson.

2   **Mt. Davidson & Saint Croix Road.** Lower stone stairway intermittently closed.

3   **Mt. Davidson Summit.** Log stairway to cross, westside.

4   **Mt. Davidson Summit.** Stone and moss stairway near cross, southside. Slippery when wet.

4   **Mt. Davidson Summit.** Stone stairway and log stairway at Saint Croix Road into forest setting and City view, across from Juanita Trail.

3   **Mt. Davidson Summit.** Stone stairway at upper Saint Croix Road.

3   **Mt. Davidson Summit.** Log and root stairways—Native Garden Trail.

4   **Mt. Davidson Summit. East Ridge Trail and Sherwood Trail at summit.** Wood stairways.

2   **Vista Verde Court at Stillings.** Wood stairway and greenery.

3   **Yerba Buena, near Maywood, to Mariloma.** Corner-cutter.

3   **Yerba Buena to Upper Yerba Buena at Ravenswood.**

NOB HILL

A famous neighborhood well-known to tourists.

RATING

2   **Clay to Washington, opposite No. 1171 Clay.** Narrow. Scavengers' access. Near Cable Car Museum.

4   **Grace Cathedral at California & Taylor.** Great stairway to cathedral.

3   **Huntington Park. California at Taylor & Cushman Alley, into park.**

3   **Huntington Park. Sacramento at Taylor & Cushman Alley, into park.**

3   **Huntington Park. Taylor/California & Sacramento, into park.**

4   **Joice Alley at Pine to Sacramento/Powell & Stockton.** Graceful curve at Pine.

2   **Mason at California.** Short sidewalk stairway.

2   **Phoenix, opposite No. 1154 Pacific/Taylor & Jones.** Dead end.

2   **Priest, opposite No. 1350 Washington.** Dead end.

2   **Reed, opposite No. 1370 Washington.** Connects to Priest Stairway.

3   **Taylor/Pine & California.** Sidewalk stairway on both sides of the street.

NOE VALLEY

An authentic neighborhood.

RATING

3   **Castro/Day & No. 500 30th St.** We have non-streets and double streets and stairways intersecting. Adjacent Franciscan rock cliffs. Entrance to Glen Park neighborhood.

4   **Castro/28th St. & Duncan.** Panoramic views. Franciscan rock formation. Wildlife haven. Strenuous walking.

3 **Cesar Chavez/Castro at No. 4220 & Diamond.** Two-level stairway with walkways.

3 **Cuesta Court to Grand View at No. 601, near 24th St.** Hidden. Nicely planted area. Stairway is under Market.

4 **Cuesta Court/Portola & Corbett.** Exceptional view. Cotoneaster and Monterey pines.

3 **Day at No. 493, up to No. 2350 Castro.** Go up.

2 **Duncan/Noe toward Sanchez.** Duncan is so steep that it is free of traffic from here to Diamond.

4 **Elizabeth/Hoffman & Grand View.** Sidewalk stairways on both sides. One of the grandest of the sidewalk stairways.

2 **Noe/Cesar Chavez & 27th St.** Sidewalk stairway.

3 **27th St. at Castro & Newberg.** Stairway atop high retaining wall.

3 **27th St./Castro & Noe, from cul-de-sac at end of 27th St. to Noe.**

2 **Valley/Castro to Noe.** Steep driveways show height of original street. Several small stairways.

3 **Valley/Diamond & Castro.** Wildlife haven. Stairways on both sides.

NORTH BEACH

A neighborhood in transition from predominantly Italian settlers to Chinese.

RATING

4 **Kearny/Vallejo & Broadway.** Total pedestrian block. Strenuous. Adjacent post–1906 houses are unfortunately disappearing.

2 **Powell at Filbert, into Washington Square Playground.**

2 **Romolo/Vallejo & Fresno, west of Kearny.**

3 **Tuscany at Lombard/Stockton & Powell.** Like the Winchester Mystery House stairs, these go nowhere.

2 **Wayne at Pacific/Mason & Powell.** Stairway at end of lane.

PACIFIC HEIGHTS

A neighborhood that has maintained standards in architecture and appearance. Enviable views and private schools.

RATING

1 **Allyne Park at Green & Gough.** Stone stairway in park garden.

3 **Alta Plaza.** Interior of park. Four stairways.

5 **Alta Plaza. Pierce at Clay, into park.** Beautifully proportioned, extremely wide, tiered. Amid low shrubbery and lawn. Designed by John McLaren.

3 **Alta Plaza. Pierce at Jackson, into park.** Sunny. View to North Bay.

5 **Alta Plaza. Scott/Clay & Washington, into park.** Elegant stairway surrounded by elaborate Victorians.

5 **Alta Plaza. Steiner/Clay & Washington, into park.** Beginning a series of wide stairs.

5 **Alta Plaza. Steiner at Washington, into park.** Imposing entrance. Benches and paths to four corners of the park.

2 **Baker/Green & Vallejo.** Sidewalk stairways on both sides of street.

5 **Baker/Vallejo & Broadway.** Plantings of Monterey pine, marguerites, and hebe. Walk on the west side and experience stair walking vs. uphill walking.

4 **Broderick/Broadway & Vallejo.** View. The configuration has changed and it can be too treacherous.

5 **Fillmore/Broadway & Green.** Sidewalk stairways on both sides of street. Spectacular views. Lower section built in 1915.

4 **Green/Scott & Pierce.** Stairway embedded in center of wide sidewalk.

3 **Lafayette Park. Gough at Clay, into park, connecting on path to tennis courts.** Adjacent to apartment building.

3 **Lafayette Park. Gough at Sacramento, into park.** Stairway originally went to house of one Holladay, a squatter! Dog-run area nearby.

3 **Lafayette Park. Gough at Washington, into park.**

2 **Lafayette Park. Interior Park.** Four stairways.

1 **Lafayette Park. Laguna at Sacramento, into park.** Steps to path.

3 **Lafayette Park. Laguna at Washington, into park.** Sunbathers in summer.

5 **Lyon/Green & Vallejo & Broadway.** Designed by Louis Upton, 1916. View. Complete arrangement of stairs, planting areas, landings.

4 **Normandie Terrace at Vallejo.** Built 1938, not accepted by the City until 1976.

3 **Octavia/Washington & Jackson.** Surrounded by mansions. Stairways within cul-de-sac. Originally was a private street.

1 **Vallejo at Lyon.** Stairs to nowhere.

3 **Vallejo/Scott & Pierce.** Sidewalk stairway.

3 **Webster/Broadway & Vallejo.** Sidewalk stairway across from Flood Mansion, which is now a private school.

PARKSIDE

A community of pluses and minuses. From sand dunes and fog, to flowers and ethnic diversity.

RATING

2   **Judah/LaPlaya & Great Highway.** Concrete stairway.

2   **McCoppin Square. 22nd Ave., near Taraval.** Stairway into square.

2   **Stern Grove. 19th Ave. & Sloat.** Multiple stairways on paths within grove.

PARNASSUS HEIGHTS

Home of University of California Medical School, with Sutro Forest, once Ishi's preserve, as the background.

RATING

2   **Belgrave, at end of street, to Tank Hill.**

1   **Belgrave, near Stanyan, into interior Park Belt.** Informal, leading upward to rough trail.

3   **Farnsworth/Edgewood & Willard.** Beautiful and meandering.

3   **Kirkham at 4th Ave., up to 1550 5th Ave., behind UC Medical School.** Wood stairway. Hidden in the woods.

3   **Stanyan, near No. 1289/Belgrave & 17th St. Stairways on both sides of street.** Formerly up to Clarendon.

PORTOLA

A neighborhood showing strains.

RATING

2   **Campus Lane/Princeton & Burrows.**

3   **Dwight/Goettingen & Hamilton.** Very long. View.

3   **Goettingen & Dwight.**

POTRERO HILL

Beautiful weather and views.

RATING

3   **Carolina/19th & 20th Sts.** Views of Bay Bridge and freeway network. Embankment plantings by Victoria Mews Association. Beautiful. Secluded.

3   **Carolina at Southern Heights.** Curved concrete stairway.

1   **Connecticut (end), up to Arkansas at 22nd St. Stwy.** Dirt path to wood plank stairway.

4   **Kansas/22nd & 21st Sts., from No. 980 to No. 965 Kansas.** Hidden. At end of two woodsy, deadend streets, upper and lower. Cobblestone brick and concrete stairs and paths. Long, zigzag, rustic gardens.

2   **Mariposa/Utah & Potrero.** Sidewalk stairway on both sides.

2   **McKinley Square.** One stairway on trail on west side of park. Great views.

3   **McKinley Square.** Several stairways within McKinley Square.

4   **McKinley Square Playground. San Bruno at 20th St., into square.** View.

3   **McKinley Square Playground. Vermont at 20th St., into square.**

2   **19th St./De Haro & Rhode Island.** Crooked dirt path and wood stairways. Can be slippery if wet.

2   **24th St./Rhode Island & De Haro.** Sidewalk stairway on both sides of street.

3   **22nd St./ Wisconsin & Connecticut, into Potrero Hill Recreation Center.** Rural. View.

2   **22nd St./Kansas & Rhode Island.** Sidewalk stairway. Very steep.

3   **23rd St./Lower Carolina & Upper Carolina.**

3   **23rd St./Carolina & Wisconsin.** Two stairways. Split, landscaped street.

4   **Vermont/20th St. to 22nd St.** Curly street. Three stairways along street radiate from successive cul-de-sacs.

PRESIDIO

Founded in 1776 by the Spanish under leaders Moraga and Anza. Obtain map of area at the Visitors' Center.

RATING

2   **Baker Beach, up to Baker Beach Road.**

3   **Baker Beach Stwy. Lincoln Blvd./Pershing Drive & Kobbe Ave. to Baker Beach.** Logs and chains. Excellent view of Golden Gate Bridge.

3   **Coastal Trail/Golden Gate Bridge & Fort Point.** Wood stairway.

2   **Coastal Trail just east of Golden Gate Bride.** Stairway up to wood viewing platform.

3   **Coastal Trail just east of Golden Gate Bridge.** Stairway down into and up out of historic brick battery tunnel.

4   **Coastal Trail, just west of Golden Gate Bridge.** Wood stairway. View.

5   **Connector Stairways. Between Park Blvd. & Cemetery Overlook; between Lincoln Blvd. & Immigrant Overlook & Rob Hill Campground.**

2   **8th Ave./Lake & Mountain Lake Park.**

2   **Golden Gate Bridge.** Stairways leading to bridge and to gift shop.

4   **Letterman Digital Arts Center. Gorgas Gate at Gorgas & Lyon.** Stone stairway into garden area near metal arches.

4   **Letterman Digital Arts Center. Park Garden/Chestnut & Francisco.** Natural stone stairway near pond; Gorgas Gate stone stairway into garden.

2   **Lincoln Blvd. at Hoffman.**

3   **MacArthur Ave., to end at El Polin Spring.** Wood stairway to path leading to Julius Kahn Playground.

3   **Moraga/Funston & Barnard.** Good for exploring.

1   **Multiple stairways at gunnery and battery sites in the Presidio.**

3   **Multiple stairways. Simonds Loop, Gibbon Ct., Infantry Terrace, Amatury Loop.** Additional stairways throughout the Presidio.

2   **Presidio Blvd. at Nos. 548–550, near MacArthur Ave./Lombard & Lincoln Blvd.** Stone stairway and three street-to-sidewalk stairways.

2   **12th Ave. at playground into Mountain Lake Park.**

1   **Young & Lincoln.**

1   **Young to Main Presidio Post, behind Crissy Field Center.**

RICHMOND

Known as the "sand waste" area in early days of San Francisco.

RATING

4   **Balboa/No. 641 48th Ave. & LaPlaya.** Wood stairway. Paths along graffiti-covered fence leading to Sutro Heights Blvd. Magnificent view of Pacific Ocean.

5   **California/32nd Ave. & golf course, to Lincoln Park.** Surrounded by cypresses. Twenty-nine-inch wide stairway with landings and benches. Footpath to the Palace of Legion of Honor.

2   **Clement/43rd and 44th Aves. up to VA Hospital.**

2   **48th Ave. & Balboa.** Cul-de-sac with sidewalk stairways on both sides.

2   **Great Hwy./Balboa & Sloat.** Multiple concrete stairways from sidewalk to beach. Can be laden with sand. Watch your footing.

4   **Lake/El Camino Del Mar to 30th Ave.** Stairways between three levels of Lake. Very pretty.

5 **Sutro Heights Park at 48th Ave./Point Lobos Ave. & Anza.** Twenty-one-acre estate of Adolph Sutro, purchased in 1881. The four separate stairways to and around the ramparts offer excellent ocean views.

4 **3rd Ave. Nos. 1–11 at Lake.** A full-sized sculpture of a cow has been watching over this stairway for many years.

RUSSIAN HILL

Grave of Russians buried on the hill account for the neighborhood name.

RATING

2 **Broadway/Jones and Taylor.** Sidewalk stairway.

1 **Broadway Tunnel West Mini Park/Cyrus & Hyde.**

1 **Broadway Tunnel East Mini Park/Himmelman Place at Broadway.**

5 **Chestnut/Polk & Larkin.** In center of Chestnut cul-de-sac. Very wide. Foliage. Double stairway up to Larkin.

3 **Culebra Terrace/No. 1250 Lombard & Chestnut.** Charming. Terraced.

5 **Filbert/Hyde & Leavenworth.** Sidewalk stairway. Coit Tower straight ahead. Strenuous walk up a 31.5% grade.

3 **Florence/Broadway & Vallejo.** Charming. Pueblo Revival houses near the 1939 stairway.

3 **Francisco/Lower Leavenworth & Francisco.** Surmounts huge retaining wall to secluded street.

5 **Francisco/Upper Leavenworth & Hyde.** Three stairways. Ivy cascading down walls, urns, and pines. View to the north.

2 **George Sterling Park at Larkin & Lombard.** Interior park.

4 **Green/Jones & Taylor, next to No. 940 Green.**

5 **Greenwich/Hyde & Larkin.** Near tennis courts.

5 **Greenwich/Hyde & Leavenworth.** View.

5 **Greenwich (south side)/Leavenworth & Jones.** Michelangelo Park. One of the most beautiful multi-use neighborhood parks in the City.

1 **Hastings/Filbert & Union.** Dead end stairway.

4 **Havens/Leavenworth & Hyde, in cul-de-sac.** Entrance only on west side of Leavenworth. Charming.

2 **Himmelman Place to Salmon.** Utilitarian, with Mini Park alongside.

1 **Houston/Jones & Columbus, next to 2430 Jones.**

3 **Hyde & Francisco.** Corner stairways on both corners. Necessary.

5 **Jones/Filbert & Union & Green.** Nicely proportioned. Raised sidewalk stairway. Hard work. Stairs have a visual pattern of horizontal louvered shades.

3 Jones—Upper to Lower Jones at Vallejo.

4 Larkin/Francisco & Bay. Long series of stairways. Pass by reservoir paths.

3 Larkin/Chestnut & Francisco, beginning at No. 2745 Larkin. View of reservoir and slope of vegetation.

5 Lombard/Hyde & Leavenworth. Curly here, straight there.

2/5 Macondray Lane/Leavenworth & Taylor. The eastern section of Macondray is Shangri-la; the western is not. At the present time, the stairway is not safe to use.

3 Montclair Terrace/Lombard & Chestnut. Hidden.

1 Redfield Alley. An interrupted alley.

3 Russian Hill Park at Bay/Hyde & Larkin. Stone stairway in park at top.

5 Vallejo/Jones & Taylor. Retaining wall dates to 1914. View. Entrance to special section of Vallejo that has historic value. Willis Polk designed houses on Russian Hill Place and stairway entrance on Jones.

5 Vallejo/Mason & Taylor. Winding.

2 Valparaiso/Filbert & Greenwich on Taylor.

ST. FRANCIS WOOD

One of the finest residential parks designed West of Twin Peaks. Developed by Mason & McDuffie between 1912 and 1918.

RATING

3 Junipero Serra to Santa Ana/Darian & Monterey. Long concrete walkway, with stairs to start.

3 Portola at Santa Clara. Across from No. 1420 Portola. West of Vicente. Near Terrace.

3 St. Francis Blvd. at San Anselmo, Upper Fountain. Stairway on each side of the plaza.

3 St. Francis Blvd. at Santa Ana, Lower Fountain. Two small stairways to fountain in center of the circle.

2 San Anselmo & Santa Ana at Portola. Corner stairway.

1 Stonestown Stwy./19th Ave. & Stonestown Center. Across from Mercy High School.

2 Terrace Drive at Terrace Walk Stwy. Down to tennis courts.

2 Terrace Drive, opposite No. 141. Down to lawn.

5 Terrace Walk/San Anselmo & Yerba Buena. Rebuilt of solid redwood, amid trees and parkland. Stairways up and down.

SEACLIFF

Beautiful ocean views; large homes. A hop and skip from Lands End hiking trails and the Palace of the Legion of Honor.

RATING

1   **China Beach.** Six stairways around structures.

3   **China Beach Road, opposite No. 455, from path to China Beach.** Wood stairway.

2   **Seacliff. North 25th Ave. in Seacliff, to Baker Beach.**

4   **Seacliff at No. 330.** Rounding a corner. In the elegant Seacliff neighborhood.

4   **Seacliff.** Multiple street-to-sidewalk stairways in this neighborhood.

4   **Seacliff. 27th Ave./Seacliff & El Camino Del Mar.** Beautiful area. Four brick stairways.

SOUTH OF MARKET

Once an early residential neighborhood—subsequently industrial, presently mixed. Changed to lofts, Giants Baseball Park, Mission Bay UC Medical Center, condos.

RATING

3   **Beale/Main & Fremont to Harrison, opposite No. 228.** Ed Beale was the first to bring gold samples to the East Coast, in 1848. On old Rincon Hill, anchor of the Bay Bridge.

3   **Bryant/1st St. & Rincon.** Near steep switchback steel-rail stairway climbing the wall near the Bay Bridge anchorage.

*   **Lansing/1st St. & Essex.** Freeway fumes with every breath. Once, in Gold Rush times, this was an elegant neighborhood.

4   **Yerba Buena Gardens/Mission & Howard, 3rd & 4th Sts.** The area, after 30 years of being a civic eyesore, has evolved into the pride of San Francisco, five and one-half acre park, galleries, butterfly gardens, outdoor sculptures, and 20-foot high waterfall.

3   **Yerba Buena Lane at 757 Market to Mission/2nd & 3rd Sts.**

SUNNYSIDE

Neighborhood worth exploring.

RATING

4   **Detroit/Joost, Monterey, & Hearst.** Very handy. A stairway crossing a main thoroughfare. Compare with Harry Stwy.

2   **Forester at Melrose, across from Sunnyside Playground.**

5   **Joost-Baden Mini-Park /Nos. 242 & 250 Joost & Nos. 149 & 151 Mangels.** Great landscaping. Views of San Bruno Mtn.

4   **Melrose Stwy./Teresita to Mangels to Sunnyside Playground.** Starts down from No. 195 Melrose. Much variety in the series. Melrose is a double street! The 800 block of Teresita is across from No. 195 Melrose.

2   **Monterey—Upper Monterey to Lower Monterey at Plymouth.**

5   **Next to No. 233 Joost, down to Monterey Blvd., via historic Sunnyside Conservatory.** Unusual landscaping designed by Ted Kipping, neighbor and arborist.

TELEGRAPH HILL

Early photographs show stairways literally hanging over the cliffs of this historic neighborhood. Three new stairways leading to Coit Tower were built in 2005.

RATING

2   **Bartol Alley at No. 379 Broadway to Vallejo.** Franciscan formation under an adjacent house.

3   **Child/Lombard & Telegraph Place.** Almost unseen. Form and function in accord.

4   **Coit Tower. Down to path (west side).**

2   **Coit Tower. Entrance (north side).**

3   **Coit Tower. Rear lawn area. Pioneer Park.** Five stairways.

4   **Coit Tower. Rear path to Telegraph Hill Blvd. (south side).**

5   **Filbert/Grant & Kearny, next to Garfield School.** Steps of perfect proportion.

3   **Filbert/Kearny & Telegraph Hill Blvd.**

5   **Filbert/Telegraph Hill Blvd. & Montgomery & Sansome.** Part of Historic District. Wonderful, extensive plantings.

4   **Francisco/Kearny & Grant.** An attractive access to Coit Tower. Wood stairway that begins in a garden setting and ends in a gardened cul-de-sac, with an unusual elevated walkway in between.

2   **Genoa Place/Filbert & Union.**

4   **Grant/Francisco & Chestnut.** Jack Early Park. An oasis for neighborhood residents and others. Perfect for moon viewing.

4   **Greenwich/Grant & Telegraph Hill Blvd.** Two stone stairways. An attractive way to the summit of the hill and Coit Tower.

5   **Greenwich/Telegraph Hill Blvd. & Montgomery & Sansome.** Unusual trees in the canyon.

3 Julius/Lombard & Whiting. Not easily seen.

1 Krausgrill at Filbert, near Stockton.

5 Lombard at Telegraph Hill Blvd., near Kearny. Stairs connect street to pathway to Coit Tower. View.

4 Montgomery/Green & Union.

3 Pardee Alley/Grant & Kramer.

2 San Antonio Place/Vallejo & Kearny.

3 Telegraph Hill Blvd. at Greenwich Stwy. (west side). Up to path to Coit Tower. Stone stairway and four donor concrete stairways.

4 Union/Calhoun & east cliff of Telegraph Hill. Close-up of geologic formation of the hill. View is an unexpected eye-opener.

1 Union at Ice House Alley/Sansome & Battery. Two small stairways.

2 Union at Sansome.

3 Vallejo/Montgomery & Kearny. Angled and tiered. Plantings throughout.

1 Vallejo at No. 474/Montgomery & Kearny.

1 Vallejo/Sansome & Battery at Cowell.

TWIN PEAKS

A focal point for the entire city, as outlined in the 1905 Burnham Beautification Report whose ideas were discarded in the mad rush to rebuild after the 1906 earthquake and fire.

RATING

2 Burnett at Hopkins to Upper Burnett to Gardenside at No. 120. Two stairways between apartments.

4 Clayton at Corbett. View. Lovely transitional stairway. Fine specimen of a corner-stairway design.

3 Clayton & Market. Graceful corner stairway.

3 Copper/Graystone & Corbett, next to No. 301 Graystone & No. 592 Corbett. Extraordinary view. Stairway in the process of disappearing.

4 Corbett at No. 670 to No. 660. Woodsy. Surprise walk.

4 Crestline at Twin Peaks Blvd. Wood stairway & trail, with spectacular views.

3 Cuesta Court, No. 42 to Corbett. Next to houses and open space.

2 Cuesta Court. Street-to-sidewalk stairway.

2 Fredela Lane/Clairview Court & Farview Court.

2 Fredela Lane/Lower Marview & Clairview Court.

2 Glendale at Corbett.

3 Iron Alley/No. 495 Corbett & No. 1499 Clayton, with an extension to Graystone. Wood stairway.

1 Market, opposite No. 3801. Dead end stairway.

1 Market/Romain & Glendale. Along sidewalk above Market.

5 Pemberton Place/Crown & Clayton. Compelling view. 1942-vintage stairway. 1995 redesign. Stamped-concrete stairway, terra-cotta color; handrails, lights. Designed by Brian Gatter. Drinking fountains for people and dogs.

5 Twin Peaks. Wood stairways up and over both peaks. Spectacular City views.

3 Twin Peaks Blvd., next to No. 192, opposite Crown Terrace up to Tank Hill. Panoramic view.

4 Twin Peaks Blvd. (Lower) to Twin Peaks Blvd. (Upper), opposite the end of Midcrest.

3 Twin Peaks at Christmas Tree Pt. Vista Area.

2 Vista Lane/Burnett at No. 535 to Gardenside to Parkridge to Crestline at No. 70. Six separate stairways with views.

UPPER MARKET

The neighborhood is enjoying a renaissance. Gardens and houses are being renovated by community groups.

RATING

2 Ashbury/No. 57 & No. 81 Ashbury Terrace. Seven small stairways between street and sidewalk.

4 Ashbury Terrace, next to No. 64. 1911–1912 development.

2 Clifford Terrace at Roosevelt No. 475, to Lower Terrace No. 180. Rounding a corner and continuing across the street.

4 Corbett, next to No. 334. Very steep alley, with stairway and walkway to 1310 Clayton.

1 Corbett & 17th St. The two steps serve the purpose of rounding the corner.

3 Corbin Place/No. 200 Corbett & No. 4399 17th St.

3 Danvers/18th St. & Market. A 1946 stairway.

3 Douglass/States & 17th St. Charming, tree-lined cul-de-sac, with an assortment of Victorians.

3 Levant/States & Roosevelt. High retaining wall covered with vines. Butterflies and chickadees abound in the foliage. Curbed street complements stairway.

3 Lower Terrace & Saturn.

1   **Ord Court at No. 2 to Douglass cul-de-sac.** Surprise.

3   **Ord/Storrie & Market, down to Ord at 18th St.** Happy wall mural on No. 176 Ord at end of stairway.

2   **Roosevelt at 17th St.** Rounding a corner.

3   **Saturn/Lower Terrace and top of Saturn Stwy.** Seven useful stairways interacting with sidewalk and street.

2   **Saturn at No. 154/Temple & Roosevelt.** One three-step stairway.

4   **Saturn/end of Saturn & Ord.** Redesigned by Department of Public Works. Benches and planted areas augment curving stairway.

2   **17th St. & Mars.** Rounding a corner.

3   **Upper Terrace. Monument Way at 17th Ave./Clayton & Roosevelt, to Upper Terrace.** View. You're at the geographical center of San Francisco.

4   **Upper Terrace. No. 480 at Mt. Olympus down to Upper Terrace No. 227.** View. Neighborly.

3   **Upper Terrace. Steps to Mt. Olympus monument.**

5   **Vulcan/Levant & Ord.** Caring neighbors and cobblestone—not to be missed.

VISITACION VALLEY

Lively mix of ethnic cultures and neighborhood participation.

RATING

3   **Beeman Lane/Wabash & San Bruno.**

3   **Campbell/San Bruno & Bayshore.**

5   **Campbell/Elliot & Visitacion Ave.** Unexpected, long, in open space setting.

3   **San Bruno to Bayshore Blvd., near Arletta.** See the inscription "Safety Subway" on the concrete wall of corner staircase.

5   **Visitacion Valley Greenway/Leland & Tioga.** Unusual setting.

2   **Ward/Girard at No. 95 & San Bruno.**

WESTERN ADDITION

This neighborhood survived the 1906 earthquake and grew and grew until it reached its peak during World War II.

RATING

3   **Alamo Square. Fulton at Pierce, into square.**

3   **Alamo Square. Fulton at Steiner, into square.**

3 **Alamo Square. Grove at Scott, into square.**

3 **Alamo Square. Grove at Steiner, into square.**

3 **Alamo Square. Hayes at Pierce, into square.**

2 **Alamo Square. Hayes/Scott & Pierce.** Divided street, four separate stairways.

4 **Cottage Row at Sutter to Bush/Webster & Fillmore.**

3 **Koshland Park. Page at Buchanan, into park.** Seven small stairways on path through park.

2 **Pierce/Duboce Park & Waller.**

2 **Steiner/Geary & Post.** Stairway to skyway over Geary.

YERBA BUENA ISLAND

Part of imperial San Francisco. Entry is first exit on the Bay Bridge traveling east.

RATING

2 **Lower Yerba Buena Road to Upper Yerba Buena Road.** Stairway and path.

3 **Macalla Court to Yerba Buena Road.** Stairways and path.

1 **Macalla Road under Bay Bridge.** Relic stairway with steel railing in the middle of nowhere.

2 **Macalla Road at Yerba Buena Road.** Connects to path along road.

2 **Yerba Buena Road at Forest Road.** Old concrete stairway to nowhere. Once connected with path to summit.

CONSERVATIVE COUNT OF STAIRWAYS

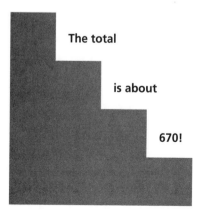

The total

is about

670!

Index

V

VA Hospital 93
Vallejo St. Crest District 42
Vallejo Stairway 13–14, 43, 44–45,
 125
van Bruggen, Coosje 213–214
Vedanta Society Temple 67
Vertigo (film) 34
Veterans Hospital 102
Victoria Mews Association 175
Victoria Park 64
Visitacion Valley Greenway 201, 202
Visitacion Valley stairways 254
Vulcan Stairway 125, 145–146

W

Wackenreuder, Vitus 176
Wade, Isabel 211
Walker, Mary 160
walks. *See also specific walk*
 gear and equipment for 3
 list of stairways 221–255
 in this book 3
Walton Square 27
Washington Square 29
Washington Square Park 22
Washington Towers 10
Wave Organ 75
Webster Historic District 70
Western Addition stairways 254–255

Weston, Edward Payson 76
Westwood Highlands 112–117
Wharf Plaza 27
What Cheer House 9
White, Dan 155
Wild Parrots of Telegraph Hill (book
 and film) xvii, 27
Wilder, Laura Ingalls 44
William Stout Architectural Books
 12
Williams, Doris 44
Woods, Corinne 211
Woodward, R. B. 9
Woolf, Virginia 140, 198, 204
Worcester, Joseph 44
Wordsworth, William 63, 173
Works Progress Administration
 (WPA) projects 14, 84

Y

Yat-sen, Sun 10
Yellin, Samuel 38
Yerba Buena Cove 5–8, 18
Yerba Buena Island stairways 255
Yoda fountain 74
Yosemite Marsh 198
Yung, Nicholas 37

Z

Zoetrope Building 13

About the Author

Adah Bakalinsky grew up in St. Paul, Minnesota, surrounded by flat land. She remembers trying, as a child, to walk up icy Ramsey Hill (near Pleasant Avenue) in winter, slithering down, trying again, and finally reaching the top. Fifty years later, while walking the old neighborhood on a visit, she discovered a stairway had been built to ascend the hill!

Looking for a synthesis for her social work, music, and film background, she discovered, surprisingly, that it was walking. She walks and, as she walks, she talks to whomever will talk with her. She carries a tape recorder to capture stories; she finds that walks shape themselves into a variety of musical forms and dances, and she

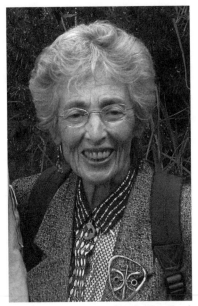

photo by Kate Brock

redesigns a walk until it has just the rhythm it must have. She walks to see and returns to photograph the objects that give flavor to the walk. She feels lucky to live in San Francisco, where walking seems the most natural way to traverse the City.

Happy heeling, frisky footing, and merry walking!

About the Team

Marian Gregoire grew up in Wisconsin and enjoyed a career as a telecommunications system design specialist. While out on a neighborhood walk in the Presidio after her retirement, she and a fellow walker decided to continue on their own but ended up talking instead. Marian explained how much she wished she'd celebrated the stairway walk day held in honor of the 20th anniversary of *Stairway Walks in San Francisco*, and her companion responded, "I'm the author of that book!"

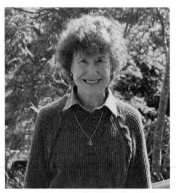

photo by Clayton Juan

Following their fortuitous meeting, Adah included Marian in her "sacred Tuesday" exploring group, who may not know exactly where they'll end up but always enjoy the adventure. On their walks Marian has learned to notice everything from flowers, plants, and trees to the architecture of a house and the use of open space. She considers her work on the sixth and seventh editions with Adah a stimulating learning experience. Best of all, they have become good friends who look forward to their continuing walks and discoveries.

Charles Brock grew up in Burlingame and retired in 2005 after more than three decades as a park ranger for the San Mateo County Parks and Recreation Department. He met Adah on a stairway that same year and subsequently shared many ideas and much legwork for the sixth and seventh editions, including the "List of Stairways." He now lives in Portland, Oregon.

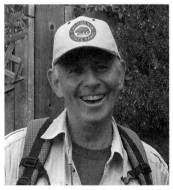

photo by Kate Brock

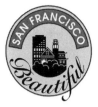

San Francisco Beautiful

San Francisco Beautiful was founded in 1947 by Friedel Klussmann in the course of her successful campaign to save the City's fabled cable cars. The organization's stated mission is to create, enhance, and protect the unique beauty and livability of San Francisco. It encourages and rewards citizen activism through its coveted annual Beautification Awards, works with civic leaders and community organizations to promote healthy and sustainable urban planning and design policies, and gives grants for neighborhood improvement projects. Preserving and restoring the City's public stairways and stairway gardens is of particular interest to the organization.

People interested in supporting San Francisco stairways and other neighborhood improvement projects, and San Francisco residents looking for assistance in improving their neighborhood stairways should visit www.sfbeautiful.org for membership, donor, and grant information.

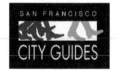

San Francisco City Guides

San Francisco City Guides is a volunteer organization that gives more than 50 free walking tours throughout the City, including walks on San Francisco stairways. Since 1978, City Guides have been leading these informative tours of San Francisco's history, architecture, legends, and lore. These tours are sponsored by the San Francisco Public Library. For more information on participating in a City Guides walk or becoming a volunteer, visit www.sfcityguides.org.